Workbook for
Hartman's Nursing Assistant Care
The Basics

FIFTH EDITION

by Hartman Publishing, Inc.

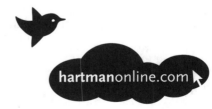
hartmanonline.com

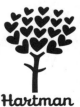
Hartman

Credits

Managing Editor
Susan Alvare Hedman

Cover Designer
Kirsten Browne

Production
Tracy Kopsachilis

Proofreaders
Sara Alexander
Sapna Desai
Joanna Owusu

Copyright Information

© 2019 by Hartman Publishing, Inc.
1313 Iron Avenue SW
Albuquerque, New Mexico 87102
(505) 291-1274
web: hartmanonline.com
e-mail: orders@hartmanonline.com
Twitter: @HartmanPub

ISBN 978-1-60425-101-2

PRINTED IN THE USA

Second Printing, 2019

Notice to Readers

Though the guidelines and procedures contained in this text are based on consultations with healthcare professionals, they should not be considered absolute recommendations. The instructor and readers should follow employer, local, state, and federal guidelines concerning healthcare practices. These guidelines change, and it is the reader's responsibility to be aware of these changes and of the policies and procedures of his or her healthcare facility.

The publisher, author, editors, and reviewers cannot accept any responsibility for errors or omissions or for any consequences from application of the information in this book and make no warranty, express or implied, with respect to the contents of the book. The publisher does not warrant or guarantee any of the products described herein or perform any analysis in connection with any of the product information contained herein.

Gender Usage

This workbook uses gender pronouns interchangeably to denote healthcare team members and residents.

Table of Contents

Preface

Welcome to the *Workbook for Nursing Assistant Care: The Basics*! This workbook is designed to help you review what you have learned from reading your textbook. For this reason, the workbook is organized around learning objectives, just like the textbook and your instructor's teaching material.

These learning objectives work as a built-in study guide. After completing the exercises for each learning objective in the workbook, ask yourself if you can *do* what that learning objective describes.

If you can, move on to the next learning objective. If you cannot, just go back to the textbook, reread that learning objective, and try again.

We have provided procedure checklists close to the end of the workbook. There is also a practice test for the certification exam. The answers to the workbook exercises are in your instructor's teaching guide.

Happy learning!

1

The Nursing Assistant in Long-Term Care

1. Compare long-term care to other healthcare settings

Multiple Choice
Circle the letter of the answer that best completes the statement or answers the question.

1. Another name for a long-term care facility is
   (A) Skilled nursing facility
   (B) Home healthcare facility
   (C) Assisted living facility
   (D) Adult day services facility

2. Assisted living facilities are initially for
   (A) People who need 24-hour skilled care
   (B) People who need some help with daily care
   (C) People who will die within six months
   (D) People who need acute care

3. Which of the following statements is true of adult day services?
   (A) This type of care is for people who need to live in the facility where the care is provided.
   (B) This type of care is for people who need some help and supervision during certain hours.
   (C) Most people who need adult day services are seriously ill or disabled.
   (D) Many types of outpatient surgeries are performed at adult day services centers.

4. Care given by specialists to restore or improve function after an illness or injury is called
   (A) Acute care
   (B) Subacute care
   (C) Rehabilitation
   (D) Hospice care

5. Care given to people who have about six months or less to live is called
   (A) Acute care
   (B) Subacute care
   (C) Rehabilitative care
   (D) Hospice care

6. People who live in long-term care facilities are usually called _____ because it is where they live for the duration of their stay.
   (A) Patients
   (B) Healthcare providers
   (C) Regulators
   (D) Residents

7. Most conditions seen in long-term care are chronic. What does this mean?
   (A) The conditions require immediate treatment at a hospital.
   (B) The conditions last a long time.
   (C) The conditions last a short time.
   (D) The conditions will usually cause death within three months.

2. Describe a typical long-term care facility

True or False
Mark each statement with either a T for true or an F for false.

1. _____ Long-term care facilities may offer assisted living, subacute care, or specialized care.

2. _____ Facilities that offer specialized care must have specially trained employees.

3. _____ Nonprofit organizations cannot own long-term care facilities.

4. _____ Person-centered care means that staff should treat all residents exactly the same.

5. _____ Culture change means basing care on each individual's needs.

3. Explain Medicare and Medicaid

Short Answer

1. List two groups of people who qualify for Medicare.

_____

_____

_____

2. List the four parts of Medicare and what each helps pay for.

_____

_____

_____

_____

_____

_____

_____

_____

_____

_____

3. How is eligibility for Medicaid determined?

_____

_____

_____

_____

4. Describe the nursing assistant's role

Short Answer

1. What are three tasks that nursing assistants are not allowed to perform?

_____

_____

_____

_____

2. What is one reason that observing and reporting changes in a resident's condition is important?

_____

_____

_____

_____

3. If a nursing assistant (NA) sees a resident who is not on his assignment sheet but who needs help, what should the NA do?

_____

_____

_____

_____

5. Describe the care team and the chain of command

Matching
Use each letter only once.

1. _____ Activities Director

2. _____ Licensed Practical Nurse (LPN) or Licensed Vocational Nurse (LVN)

3. _____ Medical Social Worker (MSW)

4. _____ Nursing Assistant (NA)

5. _____ Occupational Therapist (OT)

6. _____ Physical Therapist (PT or DPT)

7. _____ Physician or Doctor (MD or DO)

8. ____   Registered Dietitian (RD or RDN)

9. ____   Registered Nurse (RN)

10. ____   Resident

11. ____   Speech-Language Pathologist (SLP)

(A) Performs assigned tasks, such as measuring vital signs and providing personal care

(B) Diagnoses disease or disability and pre-scribes treatment

(C) Licensed professional who has completed one to two years of education and is able to administer medications and give treatments

(D) Person whose condition, treatment, and progress are the focus of the care team

(E) Gives therapy in the form of heat, cold, mas-sage, ultrasound, electrical stimulation, and exercise to muscles, bones, and joints

(F) Identifies communication disorders and cre-ates a care plan, as well as teaches exercises to help the resident improve or overcome speech problems

(G) Helps residents learn to adapt to disabilities by training them to perform activities of daily living and other activities

(H) Evaluates residents' nutritional status and develops treatment plans, including creating special diets to meet residents' needs

(I) Helps residents get support services, such as counseling

(J) Coordinates, manages, and provides skilled nursing care, as well as supervises nursing assistants' daily care of residents

(K) Plans activities to help residents socialize and stay mentally and physically active

Multiple Choice

12. Which of the following statements is true of the chain of command?
    (A) It describes the line of authority.
    (B) It is the same as the care team.
    (C) It details the survey process for each facility.
    (D) Nursing assistants are at the top of the chain of command.

13. Liability is a legal term that means
    (A) The line of authority in a facility
    (B) Ignoring a resident's call light
    (C) Someone can be held responsible for harming someone else
    (D) A task that a person is not trained for

14. Why should a nursing assistant not do tasks that are not assigned to him?
    (A) The NA may be assigned more work if he performs additional tasks.
    (B) The NA may put himself or a resident in danger.
    (C) The NA may need to pay for additional training.
    (D) The NA may have to arrive at work earlier.

15. What is one reason that other members of the care team will show great interest in the work that a nursing assistant does?
    (A) Licensed healthcare providers may not trust the NA.
    (B) Licensed healthcare providers assign the NA's tasks.
    (C) The NA will most likely sue a licensed healthcare provider if not watched carefully.
    (D) Licensed healthcare providers do not respect unlicensed healthcare personnel, like nursing assistants.

6. Define policies, procedures, and professionalism

True or False

1. ____   A policy is a course of action to be fol-lowed. For example, all health infor-mation must remain confidential.

2. ____   Facilities will have procedures for reporting information about residents.

3. ____   It is all right to do tasks not listed in the job description if they are very simple.

4. ____   Changes in a resident's condition should be reported to the nurse.

5. ____   Each step in a procedure is important and must be strictly followed.

Short Answer

Mark each of the following items with a P for professional behavior or a U for unprofessional behavior.

6. _____ Being on time for work

7. _____ Being neatly dressed and groomed

8. _____ Doing tasks that have not been assigned if the resident requests them

9. _____ Keeping resident information confidential

10. _____ Telling a resident about a bad date that the NA had over the weekend

11. _____ Explaining care before providing it

12. _____ Accepting a birthday gift from a resident

13. _____ Providing person-centered care

14. _____ Asking questions when not sure of something

15. _____ Calling a favorite resident *Sweetie*

16. _____ Being a positive role model

17. _____ Answering a call while helping a resident eat dinner

Matching

Use each letter only once.

18. _____ Compassionate

19. _____ Conscientious

20. _____ Dependable

21. _____ Empathetic

22. _____ Honest

23. _____ Patient

24. _____ Respectful

25. _____ Sympathetic

26. _____ Tactful

27. _____ Tolerant

28. _____ Unprejudiced

(A) Being caring, concerned, considerate, empathetic, and understanding

(B) Giving the same quality of care regardless of age, gender, sexual orientation, religion, race, ethnicity, or condition

(C) Being guided by a sense of right and wrong

(D) Valuing other people's individuality and treating others politely and kindly

(E) Showing sensitivity and having a sense of what is appropriate when dealing with others

(F) Being truthful

(G) Getting to work on time and doing assigned tasks skillfully

(H) Respecting others' beliefs and practices and not judging others

(I) Identifying with the feelings of others

(J) Sharing in the feelings and difficulties of others

(K) Not losing one's temper easily, not acting irritated or annoyed, not rushing residents

7. List examples of legal and ethical behavior and explain Residents' Rights

Short Answer

Read the following sentences and answer the questions.

Matt, a new nursing assistant, tells a resident that she has to wear the flowered shirt he picked out for her.

1. Which Residents' Right does this violate?

_____

_____

_____

_____

Margaret, a nursing assistant, tells her best friend, "Ms. Picadilly's cancer is getting worse. I heard her moaning all night last night."

2. Which Residents' Right does this violate?

_____

_____

_____

_____

Harry, a nursing assistant, is measuring a resident's vital signs when the resident's family arrives. He tells them, "You'll have to come back another day. I'm busy with her right now."

3. Which Residents' Right does this violate?

_____

_____

_____

_____

Yvonne, a nursing assistant, is going off duty. Leaving Ms. Scott's room, she notices a pretty necklace. She decides to borrow it for the night, promising to herself to return it tomorrow. She knows Ms. Scott has Alzheimer's disease and will not notice that it is gone anyway.

4. Which Residents' Right does this violate?

_____

_____

_____

_____

Jane is explaining a care procedure to Mrs. Gonzalez in English. Mrs. Gonzalez only speaks Spanish. When she is finished, Jane asks Mrs. Gonzalez if she understands the procedure. Mrs. Gonzalez looks confused and does not respond. Jane begins to perform the care on Mrs. Gonzalez.

5. Which Residents' Right does this violate?

_____

_____

_____

_____

Multiple Choice

Read each of the following scenarios. Decide which of the Residents' Rights is being violated in each, and circle the correct letter.

6. Mrs. Perkins is a resident who has a visual impairment. She has misplaced her eyeglasses many times. She gets upset during eye examinations, so the staff at her facility often allow her to go without glasses for a few weeks before having them replaced. Which Residents' Right is being violated?
    (A) Services and activities to maintain a high level of wellness
    (B) The right to complain
    (C) The right to make independent choices
    (D) The right to privacy and confidentiality

7. Mr. Gallerano has a stomach ulcer that causes him minor pain. He has medication for it, but he says that it makes him nauseated and he does not want to take it. Lila, a nursing assistant, tells him that he may not have his dinner until he takes the medication. Which Residents' Right is being violated?
    (A) The right to be fully informed about rights and services
    (B) The right to participate in their own care
    (C) The right to security of possessions
    (D) The right to privacy and confidentiality

8. Ms. Mayes, a resident with severe arthritis, has a blue sweater that she loves to wear. The buttons are very tiny, and she cannot button them herself. Jim, a nursing assistant, tells her that she cannot wear the sweater today because it takes him too long to help her into it. Which Residents' Right is being violated?
    (A) The right to make independent choices
    (B) The right to participate in their own care
    (C) The right to be fully informed about rights and services
    (D) The right to privacy and confidentiality

9. Amy is a nursing assistant at Sweetwater Retirement Home. Every night when she goes home, she tells her family touching stories about the residents with whom she is working. Which Residents' Right is being violated?
    (A) The right to be fully informed about rights and services
    (B) The right to participate in their own care
    (C) The right to make independent choices
    (D) The right to privacy and confidentiality

Name: _____

10. Laura, a nursing assistant at Great Oak Extended Care Facility, is running behind with her work for the evening. She is helping Mr. Young, a resident with Alzheimer's disease, with his dinner. She is getting frustrated with him because he keeps taking the fork out of her hand and dropping it on the floor. Finally she slaps his hand to get him to stop. Which Residents' Right is being violated?
    (A) The right to security of possessions
    (B) The right to complain
    (C) The right to dignity, respect, and freedom
    (D) The right to visits

11. Ms. Land, an elderly resident, gets into a loud argument with another resident during a card game. When her daughter comes to see her later that day, Anne, an NA, tells her that Ms. Land is in a bad mood and cannot see anyone. Which Residents' Right is being violated?
    (A) The right to security of possessions
    (B) Transfer and discharge rights
    (C) The right to make independent choices
    (D) The right to visits

12. During dinner, Pete, a nursing assistant, spills hot soup on a resident's arm. He tells her that she had better not tell anyone about it or he will be very angry at her. Which Residents' Right is being violated?
    (A) The right to security of possessions
    (B) Transfer and discharge rights
    (C) The right to visits
    (D) The right to complain

Matching
Use each letter only once.

13. _____ Abuse

14. _____ Active neglect

15. _____ Assault

16. _____ Battery

17. _____ Domestic violence

18. _____ False imprisonment

19. _____ Financial abuse

20. _____ Involuntary seclusion

21. _____ Malpractice

22. _____ Negligence

23. _____ Passive neglect

24. _____ Physical abuse

25. _____ Psychological abuse

26. _____ Sexual abuse

27. _____ Sexual harassment

28. _____ Substance abuse

29. _____ Verbal abuse

30. _____ Workplace violence

(A) Actions, or the failure to act or provide proper care, resulting in unintended injury to a person

(B) The repeated use of legal or illegal drugs, cigarettes, or alcohol in a way that harms oneself or others

(C) Any unwelcome sexual advance or behavior that creates an intimidating, hostile, or offensive work environment

(D) The purposeful failure to give needed care, resulting in harm to a person

(E) The separation of a person from others against the person's will

(F) Verbal, physical, or sexual abuse of staff by other staff members or residents

(G) The intentional touching of a person without her consent

(H) A threat resulting in a person feeling fearful that he will be harmed

(I) The improper or illegal use of a person's money, possessions, property, or other assets

(J) The forcing of a person to perform or participate in sexual acts

(K) The use of spoken or written words, pictures, or gestures that threaten, embarrass, or insult a person

(L) Emotional harm caused by threatening, scaring, humiliating, intimidating, isolating, or insulting a person, or by treating him or her as a child

(M) Physical, sexual, or emotional abuse by spouses, intimate partners, or family members

(N) Purposeful mistreatment that causes physical, mental, or emotional pain or injury to someone

(O) Any treatment, intentional or unintentional, that causes harm to a person's body—includes slapping, bruising, cutting, burning, physically restraining, pushing, shoving, and rough handling

(P) The unintentional failure to provide needed care, resulting in physical, mental, or emotional harm to a person

(Q) Unlawful restraint that affects a person's freedom of movement

(R) Injury caused by professional misconduct through negligence, carelessness, or lack of skill

Short Answer

31. If a resident wants to make a complaint of abuse, what must a nursing assistant do?

_____

_____

_____

_____

_____

_____

_____

_____

Multiple Choice

32. One task of an ombudsman is to
   (A) Decide which special diet is right for a resident
   (B) Investigate and resolve resident complaints
   (C) Diagnose disease and prescribe medication
   (D) Check a resident's vital signs and report to the nurse

33. What is the purpose of the Health Insurance Portability and Accountability Act (HIPAA)?
   (A) To monitor quality of care in facilities
   (B) To protect and secure the privacy of health information
   (C) To reduce instances of abuse in facilities
   (D) To provide health insurance for uninsured elderly people

34. What is included under protected health information (PHI)?
   (A) Patient's favorite food
   (B) Patient's favorite color
   (C) Patient's social security number
   (D) Patient's library card number

35. What is the correct response by an NA if someone who is not directly involved with a resident's care asks for a resident's PHI?
   (A) Give the person the information
   (B) Ask the resident if the person may have the information
   (C) Ask the person to send a written request for the information to the resident
   (D) Tell the person that the information is confidential and cannot be given out

36. Which of the following is one way to keep private health information confidential?
   (A) Only making comments about residents on Twitter
   (B) Discussing residents' progress with a coworker in a restaurant
   (C) Using confidential rooms for reporting on residents
   (D) Only discussing residents' conditions with trusted family members

8. Explain legal aspects of the resident's medical record

Multiple Choice

1. Which of the following is true of a resident's medical chart?
   (A) A medical chart is the legal record of a resident's care.
   (B) Not all care needs to be documented.
   (C) Documentation can be put off until the next day if an NA is busy.
   (D) Medical charts are not considered legal documents.

2. When should care be documented?
   (A) Before care is given
   (B) Immediately after care is given
   (C) At the end of the day
   (D) Whenever there is time

Short Answer

Convert the following times to military time.

3. 2:10 p.m. _____

4. 4:30 a.m. _____

5. 10:00 a.m. _____

6. 8:25 p.m. _____

Convert the following times to regular time.

7. 0600 _____

8. 2320 _____

9. 1927 _____

10. 1800 _____

9. Explain the Minimum Data Set (MDS)

Short Answer

1. How does a nursing assistant's reporting affect the MDS?

   _____

   _____

   _____

   _____

   _____

   _____

2. How soon after a resident is admitted does an MDS need to be completed by a nurse?

   _____

   _____

   _____

10. Discuss incident reports

Multiple Choice

1. An incident is
   (A) An accident or unexpected event in the course of care
   (B) Any interaction between residents and staff
   (C) A normal part of facility routines
   (D) Any event in a resident's day

2. Which of the following would be considered an incident?
   (A) A resident complains of a headache.
   (B) A resident on a low-sodium diet receives and eats a regular, non-restricted meal.
   (C) A resident wants to watch TV in the common living area.
   (D) A resident needs to be transferred from his bed to a chair.

3. Incidents should be reported to
   (A) The resident's family
   (B) The charge nurse
   (C) All staff on duty at the time of the incident
   (D) The doctor on call

True or False

4. ____ Documentation of incidents helps protect the resident, the employer, and individual staff members.

5. ____ The information in an incident report is confidential.

6. ____ If an NA does not actually see an incident but arrives after it has already occurred, he should document what he thinks happened.

7. ____ The documentation of an incident should include who the NA thinks could be responsible for the incident.

8. ____ Incident reports should be factual.

9. ____ If a resident falls but is okay after the fall, an incident report does not need to be completed.

10. ____ If an NA receives an injury on the job, he should file an incident report.

2

Foundations of Resident Care

1. Understand the importance of verbal and written communications

Multiple Choice

1. Which of the following is an example of non-verbal communication?
    (A) Asking for a cup of water
    (B) Pointing to a cup of water
    (C) Screaming for a cup of water
    (D) Saying, "I do not like water."

2. Verbal communication includes
    (A) Facial expressions
    (B) Nodding one's head
    (C) Speaking
    (D) Shrugging one's shoulders

3. Nonverbal communication includes
    (A) Speaking
    (B) Facial expressions
    (C) Yelling
    (D) Oral reports

Short Answer
For each of the following, decide whether it is an objective observation (the nursing assistant [NA] can see, hear, smell, or touch it) or subjective observation (the resident must tell the NA about it). Write an O for objective and an S for subjective.

4. _____ Skin rash

5. _____ Crying

6. _____ Rapid pulse

7. _____ Headache

8. _____ Nausea

9. _____ Vomiting

10. _____ Swelling

11. _____ Cloudy urine

12. _____ Feeling sad

13. _____ Red area on skin

14. _____ Fever

15. _____ Dizziness

16. _____ Wheezing

17. _____ Chest pain

18. _____ Toothache

19. _____ Coughing

20. _____ Fruity breath

21. _____ Itchy arm

Labeling
Looking at the diagram, list examples of observations using each sense.

Smell: _____

Sight: _____

Hearing: _____

Touch: _____

Short Answer

22. What is a root?

_____

_____

23. What is a prefix?

_____

_____

24. What is a suffix?

_____

_____

25. Why should nursing assistants use simple, non-medical terms when speaking with residents and their families?

_____

_____

_____

_____

26. Where should call lights be placed in residents' rooms?

_____

_____

_____

2. Describe barriers to communication

Crossword

Across

3. Type of terminology that may not be understood by residents or their families; NAs should avoid this and speak in simple, everyday words

5. Types of questions that should be asked because they elicit more than a "yes" or "no" answer

7. Phrases used over and over again that do not really mean anything

Down

1. Type of language that, along with gestures and facial expressions, is part of nonverbal communication; NAs should be aware of this when speaking

2. Being this way and taking time to listen when residents are difficult to understand helps promote better communication

4. NAs cannot offer opinions or give this because it is not within their scope of practice

6. Asking this should be avoided when residents make statements because it often makes people feel defensive

8. Along with profanity, these types of words should not be used by NAs

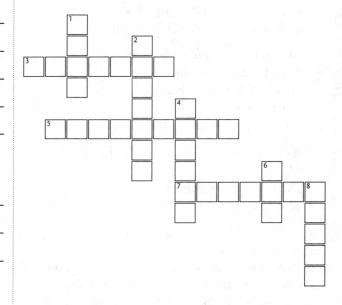

3. List guidelines for communicating with residents with special needs

Short Answer

Mark, a nursing assistant, is about to provide care for a resident who is hearing impaired. The resident is standing at the window looking out at the gardens. Mark enters her room and asks if she would like her hair shampooed. She does not answer. He taps her on the back, and she jumps. He asks loudly, "Would you like to have your hair shampooed now?"

1. What would have been a better way for Mark to communicate?

_____

_____

_____

_____

_____

_____

_____

_____

Ms. Crawford has a visual impairment. She is being helped into a fellow resident's room for a visit. Virginia, a nursing assistant, assists her to the door and says, "See you later, Ms. Crawford. I'll be back in about an hour to help you return to your room." Ms. Crawford enters the room, walks into a chair, and almost falls over.

2. What would have been a better way for Virginia to communicate with Ms. Crawford?

_____

_____

_____

_____

_____

_____

_____

Sabrina, a nursing assistant, is taking care of a resident who has a mental health disorder and is very withdrawn. Sabrina moves around the room picking up clutter and saying to her resident in a bored tone: "How are we doing today, Mrs. Rogers? Are we going to start talking to Sabrina today, or are we going to be quiet like we were yesterday?"

3. What is wrong with how Sabrina is communicating with Mrs. Rogers?

_____

_____

_____

_____

_____

_____

Resident Joe Morteno has dementia and can be combative at times. On this particular day he yells at Serena, his nursing assistant, "Why are you so stupid? You never understand what I really need!" Serena replies, "I'm not stupid! *You* don't understand what *you* need because you have dementia." She then leaves the room and tries to laugh it off.

4. What would have been a better way for Serena to communicate with Mr. Morteno?

_____

_____

_____

_____

_____

_____

Resident Hannah Singer has Alzheimer's disease. One morning Joan, a nursing assistant, sees Mrs. Singer touching herself in the hallway. Joan snaps, "Stop that right now! You are embarrassing yourself!"

5. What would have been a better way for Joan to respond to this behavior?

_____

_____

_____

Name: _____

_____
_____
_____
_____
_____

4. Identify ways to promote safety and handle non-medical emergencies

Short Answer

1. Looking at the illustrations below, which drawing (A or B) shows the correct way to lift objects? Why is it correct?

    _____
    _____
    _____
    _____
    _____
    _____
    _____
    _____
    _____

A.   B.

2. Why should an NA arrange a signal, such as counting to three, when moving a resident?

    _____
    _____
    _____
    _____
    _____

True or False

3. ____ Using proper body mechanics can help save energy and prevent injury.

4. ____ To avoid choking, residents should eat in a reclined position.

5. ____ When lifting an object, it is safer to hold it far away from the body.

6. ____ Knees should be bent when lifting an object.

7. ____ Liquids thickened to the consistency of honey are easier to swallow.

8. ____ To help guard against falls, all walkways should be cleared of clutter.

9. ____ Feet should be pointed toward the object that a person is lifting.

10. ____ A high center of gravity gives a more stable base of support.

11. ____ Keeping the feet close together gives the body the best base of support and keeps a person more stable.

12. ____ If a resident starts to fall, the nursing assistant should try to catch the resident to stop the fall.

13. ____ Residents in wheelchairs should be facing the back of the elevator when riding in elevators.

14. ____ A nursing assistant should check the temperature of hot water with a bath thermometer before using the water.

15. ____ Keeping call lights within a resident's reach can help prevent falls.

16. ____ Cuts most often occur in a person's bedroom.

17. ____ Hot drinks should be placed on the edges of tables.

18. ____ Residents must be identified before helping with feeding or placing meal trays.

19. ____ The Safety Data Sheet (SDS) details chemical ingredients and chemical dangers of products.

20. _____ A nursing assistant should call a resident by name as a way to identify the resident.

21. _____ The correct way to move a wheelchair is for a nursing assistant to push it forward.

Multiple Choice

22. If a fire occurs, a nursing assistant should
    (A) Get into the closest elevator to get to the ground floor
    (B) Block doors and windows with equipment to prevent fire from entering
    (C) Plug doorways to prevent smoke from entering
    (D) Climb up to the highest point in the room to wait for help

23. What is an NA's first concern if a fire occurs?
    (A) Getting residents to safety
    (B) Putting out the fire
    (C) Saving important documentation
    (D) Saving expensive equipment

Short Answer

24. PASS is an acronym that stands for

P: _____

A: _____

S: _____

S: _____

25. RACE is an acronym that stands for

R: _____

A: _____

C: _____

E: _____

26. Explain the fire safety technique *stop, drop, and roll.*

_____

_____

_____

_____

_____

27. What guidelines apply in any disaster situation?

_____

_____

_____

_____

_____

_____

_____

5. Demonstrate how to recognize and respond to medical emergencies

Short Answer

1. When coming upon an emergency situation, what two important steps should the NA take first?

_____

_____

_____

_____

Multiple Choice

2. First aid refers to
    (A) Care given by the first people to respond to an emergency
    (B) The person with the highest level of medical training who responds to an emergency
    (C) Any person to whom the victim has given permission for treatment during an emergency
    (D) The first person to give consent to medical professionals for treatment

3. If an emergency occurs, the NA should immediately notify the
    (A) Resident's family
    (B) Nurse
    (C) Resident's friends in the facility
    (D) Resident's clergyperson

4. How can someone usually tell if a person is choking?
(A) The choking victim will tell the person.
(B) The choking victim will ask for food.
(C) The choking victim will put his hands to his throat.
(D) The choking victim will throw up.

5. Where should the hands be placed to give abdominal thrusts?
(A) Under the person's arms and around his waist
(B) Under the person's arms and around his chest
(C) Over the person's shoulders and around his neck
(D) Under the person's arms and around his pelvis

6. How does a rescuer obtain consent to give a choking victim abdominal thrusts?
(A) The rescuer asks the victim's spouse to sign a consent form.
(B) The rescuer asks the facility administrator, "May I treat this resident who lives at your facility?"
(C) The rescuer asks his coworker.
(D) The rescuer asks the victim, "Are you choking?"

7. Signs of shock include
(A) Pale or bluish skin
(B) Lack of thirst
(C) Being asleep
(D) Relaxation

8. If an NA suspects that a resident is having a heart attack, she should
(A) Give the resident something to drink
(B) Loosen the clothing around the resident's neck
(C) Encourage the resident to walk around
(D) Leave the resident alone to rest

9. To control bleeding, an NA should
(A) Use her bare hands to stop it
(B) Lower the wound below the level of the heart
(C) Hold a thick sterile pad against the wound and press down hard
(D) Give the resident an aspirin, which will slow or stop the bleeding

10. To treat a minor burn, the NA should use
(A) Antibacterial ointment
(B) Grease, such as butter
(C) Ice water
(D) Cool, clean water

11. If a resident faints, the NA should
(A) Lower the resident to the floor
(B) Position the resident on his side
(C) Perform CPR right away
(D) Help the resident stand up immediately

12. When a resident is first experiencing signs of insulin reaction, what needs to happen?
(A) Food that can be rapidly absorbed or a glucose tablet should be consumed.
(B) The person should lie down and be left alone to rest.
(C) The nursing assistant should give the resident his diabetes medication.
(D) CPR measures should be started.

13. Which of the following is true about assisting a resident who is having a seizure?
(A) The NA should give the resident something hard to bite down on.
(B) The NA should hold the resident down if he is shaking severely.
(C) The NA should move furniture away to prevent injury to the resident.
(D) The NA should open the resident's mouth and move the tongue to one side.

14. Why is a quick response to a suspected stroke/CVA critical?
(A) A quick response means that the facility will not be liable.
(B) Early treatment may reduce the severity of the stroke.
(C) Residents will be able to say their goodbyes to loved ones.
(D) Residents will experience no side effects at all if there is a quick response.

6. Describe and demonstrate infection prevention and control practices

Multiple Choice

1. An NA will come into contact with microorganisms
   (A) Only when handling bedpans
   (B) Only by breathing close to infected residents
   (C) Only when bathing residents
   (D) Every time the NA touches something

2. The Centers for Disease Control and Prevention (CDC) defines hand hygiene as
   (A) Handwashing with soap and water or using alcohol-based hand rubs
   (B) Using alcohol-based hand rubs when hands are visibly soiled
   (C) Rinsing hands with cold water
   (D) Not washing hands more than once per day

3. Standard Precautions include the following measures:
   (A) Washing hands after taking off gloves but not before putting on gloves
   (B) Wearing gloves if there is a possibility of coming into contact with blood or body fluids
   (C) Touching body fluids with bare hands
   (D) Disposing of sharps in plastic bags

4. Why should an NA not wear artificial nails to work?
   (A) Residents may not like them.
   (B) They may be damaged during resident care.
   (C) They harbor bacteria and increase risk of contamination.
   (D) They may be torn or damaged by frequent handwashing.

5. Standard Precautions should be practiced
   (A) Only on people who look like they have a bloodborne disease
   (B) On every single person under a nursing assistant's care
   (C) Only on people who request that the nursing assistant practice them
   (D) Only on people who have tuberculosis

6. Infections acquired in healthcare settings are called
   (A) Healthcare-associated infections (HAIs)
   (B) Chains of infection (CIs)
   (C) Microorganism infections (MOIs)
   (D) Localized infections (LIs)

7. The following are links in the chain of infection. Which link is broken by wearing gloves, thus preventing the spread of disease?
   (A) Reservoir (place where the pathogen lives and grows)
   (B) Mode of transmission (a way for the disease to spread)
   (C) Susceptible host (person who is likely to get the disease)
   (D) Portal of exit (body opening that allows pathogens to leave)

8. The following are links in the chain of infection. By getting a vaccination for hepatitis B, which link will be affected to prevent a person from getting this disease?
   (A) Reservoir (place where the pathogen lives and grows)
   (B) Mode of transmission (a way for the disease to spread)
   (C) Susceptible host (person who is likely to get the disease)
   (D) Portal of exit (body opening that allows pathogens to leave)

9. How many times can disposable equipment be used before it needs to be discarded?
   (A) Three times
   (B) One time
   (C) Two times if it is washed in between uses
   (D) Indefinitely if it is sterilized in between uses

10. How should sharps, such as needles, be discarded?
    (A) Sharps should be placed in blue recycling containers.
    (B) Sharps should be placed in break room trash containers.
    (C) Sharps should be placed inside used gloves and then put in trash receptacles.
    (D) Sharps should be placed in biohazard containers.

Name: _____

11. How long should an NA use friction when lathering and washing his hands?
    (A) 2 minutes
    (B) 5 seconds
    (C) 18 seconds
    (D) 20 seconds

12. How should dirty linen be rolled or folded?
    (A) The dirty area should be inside.
    (B) The clean area should be inside.
    (C) The dirty area should be on top.
    (D) The clean area should be tucked underneath the dirty area.

13. Dirty linen should be
    (A) Shaken to remove contaminants before taking it to the soiled linen room
    (B) Carried away from the NA's uniform
    (C) Bagged outside of the resident's room
    (D) Stored in the same area as clean linen

14. Transmission-Based Precautions are used
    (A) With every resident under an NA's care
    (B) In addition to Standard Precautions
    (C) Instead of Standard Precautions
    (D) When an NA decides that they are appropriate for particular residents

15. Dedicated equipment refers to
    (A) Equipment that is used by multiple residents
    (B) Equipment donated to one resident by another resident and/or his family
    (C) Equipment that is disposable
    (D) Equipment that is used by only one resident

16. Which of the following is true of wearing personal protective equipment (PPE) while caring for residents in isolation?
    (A) Nursing assistants will have to decide for themselves which PPE they must wear while caring for residents in isolation.
    (B) Nursing assistants should remove PPE before exiting a resident's room.
    (C) Nursing assistants will always wear the same PPE while caring for all residents in isolation.
    (D) Nursing assistants should remove PPE after exiting a resident's room.

17. Bloodborne diseases can be transmitted by
    (A) Infected blood entering the bloodstream
    (B) Hugging a person with a bloodborne disease
    (C) Being in the same room as a person with a bloodborne disease
    (D) Talking to a person with a bloodborne disease

18. In health care, the most common way to get a bloodborne disease is by
    (A) Contact with infected blood or certain body fluids
    (B) Sharing contaminated needles between residents
    (C) Being in the same room as a resident with a bloodborne disease
    (D) Sexual contact with an infected resident

19. Employers must offer a free vaccine to protect NAs from
    (A) AIDS
    (B) Hepatitis B
    (C) Hepatitis C
    (D) All bloodborne diseases

20. Which of the following is true of hepatitis B (HBV)?
    (A) HBV is caused by fecal-oral contamination.
    (B) There is no vaccine for HBV.
    (C) HBV is caused by jaundice.
    (D) HBV can be transmitted through blood or needles that are contaminated with the virus.

21. Tuberculosis is
    (A) A bloodborne disease
    (B) An airborne disease
    (C) A non-infectious disease
    (D) An untreatable disease

Short Answer
Make a check mark (✓) next to the tasks that require a nursing assistant to wear gloves.

22. _____ Contact with body fluids

23. _____ When the NA may touch blood

24. _____ Brushing a resident's hair

25. _____ Answering the telephone

Foundations of Resident Care

26. _____ Assisting with perineal care

27. _____ Washing vegetables

28. _____ Giving a massage to a resident who has acne on her back

29. _____ Assisting with mouth care

30. _____ Shaving a resident

31. What is the correct order for donning (putting on) PPE (wash hands, gloves, mask, gown, goggles)?

1st _____

2nd_____

3rd _____

4th _____

5th _____

32. What is the correct order for doffing (removing) PPE (wash hands, gloves, mask, gown, goggles)?

1st _____

2nd_____

3rd _____

4th _____

5th _____

True or False

33. _____ Sterilization is a cleaning measure that destroys only pathogens, but not all microorganisms.

34. _____ Methicillin-resistant *Staphylococcus aureus* (MRSA) can be spread through indirect contact by touching objects contaminated by a person who has MRSA.

35. _____ A nursing assistant does not need to wear gloves to clean up a small spill.

36. _____ Increasing the use of antibiotics helps lower the risk of developing *Clostridium difficile* (*C. difficile*) diarrhea.

37. _____ A nursing assistant should use her hands to pick up large pieces of broken glass and use a broom and dustpan for smaller pieces.

38. _____ MRSA is almost always spread by direct physical contact.

39. _____ Handwashing will not help control the spread of MRSA.

40. _____ Vancomycin-resistant *Enterococcus* (VRE) causes life-threatening infections in people with weak immune systems.

41. _____ Frequent handwashing can help prevent the spread of VRE.

42. _____ Both hand sanitizers and washing hands with soap and water are considered equally effective when dealing with *C. difficile*.

43. _____ Disinfectant should be placed on spilled fluid before absorbing and removing the fluid.

Short Answer

Read the following and mark ER for employer or EE for employee to show who is responsible for infection prevention measures.

44. _____ Immediately report any exposure to infection, blood, or body fluids.

45. _____ Provide personal protective equipment for use, and train how to properly use it.

46. _____ Follow all facility policies and procedures.

47. _____ Take advantage of the free hepatitis B vaccination.

48. _____ Provide continuing in-service education about infection prevention.

49. _____ Establish infection prevention procedures and an exposure control plan.

50. _____ Follow resident care plans and assignments.

51. _____ Participate in annual education programs covering infection prevention.

52. _____ Use provided personal protective equipment as indicated or as appropriate.

53. _____ Provide free hepatitis B vaccinations.

Name: _____

3

Understanding Residents

1. Identify basic human needs

Short Answer

1. List five basic physical needs that all humans have.
   - Food/water
   - protection/shelter
   - sleep/rest
   - comfort
   - activity

2. List six psychosocial needs that humans have.
   - love/affection
   - acceptance
   - safety/security
   - independence
   - contact w/others
   - success & self esteem

3. Using Maslow's Hierarchy of Needs below, complete your own hierarchy of needs. The first two examples have already been completed for you.

Maslow's Hierarchy of Needs

Needs

(A) Need for self-actualization

(B) Need for self-esteem

(C) Need for love

(D) Safety and security needs

(E) Physical needs

Example of Each Need

(A) I need the chance to learn new things.

(B) I need to know that I am doing a good job.

(C) I need to know others care about me

(D) I need to know I'm safe

(E) I need food/water/sleep

True or False

4. _F_ Elderly people do not have sexual urges.

5. _T_ The ability to engage in sexual activity continues unless disease or injury occurs.

6. _T_ Residents have the legal right to choose how to express their sexuality.

7. _F_ All elderly people have the same sexual behavior and desires.

8. _T_ A nursing assistant (NA) must respect each resident's sexual orientation and gender identity.

9. _T_ The NA should always knock and wait for a response before entering residents' rooms.

10. _F_ If an NA sees a sexual encounter between consenting adult residents, she should ask them to stop.

11. _T_ If an NA encounters a resident being sexually abused, he should take the resident to a safe place and then notify the nurse.

Short Answer

Place a check mark (✓) next to examples of appropriate ways to help residents with their spiritual needs.

12. ✓ A resident tells his nursing assistant that he cannot drink milk with his hamburger due to his religious beliefs. He asks for some water instead. The NA takes the milk away and brings him water.

13. _____ A resident tells her NA that she is a Baptist and wants to know when the next Baptist service will be. The NA asks, "Why don't you just attend a Catholic service instead? I'm Catholic, and my church is close by."

14. ✓ A resident asks an NA to read a passage from his Bible. The NA opens the Bible and begins to read.

15. ✓ A resident wants to see a rabbi. The NA reports this request to the nurse.

16. _____ A nursing assistant sees a Buddha statue in a resident's room. The NA chuckles and tells the resident, "This little guy is so cute."

17. ✓ A spiritual leader is visiting with a resident. The NA quietly leaves the room and shuts the door.

18. _____ A resident tells his nursing assistant that he is Muslim. The NA begins to explain Christianity to him and asks him to attend a Christian service just to see what it is like.

19. ✓ A resident tells a nursing assistant that she does not believe in God. The NA does believe in God but does not argue with the resident. The NA listens quietly as the resident explains her reasons.

2. Define *holistic care*

Short Answer

In your own words, briefly define *holistic care*.

Taking care of the whole person, not just individual parts, but both physically & mentally.

3. Explain why promoting independence and self-care is important

Fill in the Blank

1. A loss of *independence* is very difficult for a person to deal with.

2. A nursing assistant should allow a resident to do a *possible task* independently even if it is easier for the NA to do it.

3. *activities* of daily living (ADLs) are personal care tasks a person does every day to care for himself.

4. NAs should encourage *self care*, regardless of how long it takes or how well residents are able to do it.

5. A loss of independence can cause increased *dependence*.

Case Study

Read the following scenario and answer the question below.

Sarah, a nursing assistant, is assisting Mrs. Sanchez today. It is time to get Mrs. Sanchez dressed and ready for breakfast. Sarah enters the room without knocking. She does not see Mrs. Sanchez, so she walks over to the bathroom door and opens it. Mrs. Sanchez is pulling up her underpants. "Let's go," says Sarah. "We've got to get you dressed."

Sarah chooses clean clothes and lays them out on the bed. Mrs. Sanchez starts to take off her nightgown but has trouble getting it over her head. Sarah reaches over and pulls it over her head. "Please sit down. I can do this faster."

She quickly starts putting a clean shirt on Mrs. Sanchez.

6. List all of the ways in which Sarah did NOT promote privacy, dignity, and independence.

- She did not knock or gain permission to enter the room or bathroom
- did not ask her to pick out her clothes
- did not ask if she wants help getting dressed
- touches her w/out asking

Short Answer

7. Write a brief paragraph explaining everything you did this morning before arriving at class. Include things such as bathing, using the toilet, applying makeup, fixing breakfast, brushing your hair, brushing your teeth, reading, walking around your house, etc.

- drank coffee
- ate cereal
- walked to the kitchen
- walked to the bathroom
- went pee
- brushed hair
- brushed teeth
- put on make-up
- got dressed
- packed lunch
- packed supplies for the day
- got shoes on
- put on mask
- put on shoes

8. How would you feel if you were unable to do one or more of these tasks by yourself?

- angry
- burdensome
- useless

4. Identify ways to accommodate cultural differences

Short Answer

1. Describe two examples of how you can respect and value each person as an individual.

- Remember residences' preferences for care
- remember residences' cultures/religious beliefs/ personal things about them

2. What are some things that you can do to improve your awareness of your residents' cultures and needs?

* ask Residents questions

* do research

_____

_____

_____

_____

5. Describe the need for activity

Crossword
Across

3. A type of cancer that regular physical activity lessens the risk of

5. Type of infection that inactivity can result in

6. The ability to cope with this is one benefit of regular activity

Down

1. Before activities begin, something that nursing assistants can help residents with

2. Something increased by regular activity; also promotes better eating habits

4. Abbreviation for federal law requiring that facilities provide an activities program that meets the interests of residents

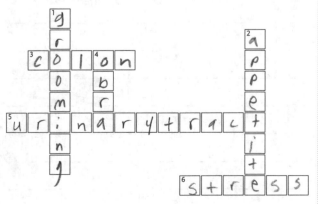

6. Discuss family roles and their significance in health care

Multiple Choice
Read each description below. Choose the term that best defines the type of family that is being described.

1. Mr. Dane's wife died giving birth to their twin girls. Mr. Dane never remarried and raised the girls himself.
    (A) Single-parent family
    (B) Nuclear family
    (C) Blended family
    (D) Extended family

2. Ms. Cone has lived with her best friend, Ms. Lawrence, since they graduated from college together. They both dated men throughout their lives but were never married. Ms. Cone has a teenage daughter who was raised in their household.
    (A) Single-parent family
    (B) Nuclear family
    (C) Blended family
    (D) Extended family

3. Mrs. Rose had three children with her first husband. She divorced him when their youngest child was two years old. Two years later she remarried, and she and her second husband raised her three children as well as one child from his first marriage.
    (A) Single-parent family
    (B) Nuclear family
    (C) Blended family
    (D) Extended family

4. Mrs. Parker was married to her husband for 30 years. They lived together with their two children.
    (A) Single-parent family
    (B) Nuclear family
    (C) Blended family
    (D) Extended family

5. Mr. Potter was married in his twenties. He and his wife moved in with her parents and had three children. After his younger sister got divorced, she also moved in with them.
    (A) Single-parent family
    (B) Nuclear family
    (C) Blended family
    (D) Extended family

6. Mr. Barter and Mr. Singer have been in a committed relationship for 15 years. They live with their 10-year-old daughter.
    (A) Single-parent family
    (B) Nuclear family
    (C) Blended family
    (D) Extended family

7. How are families now defined?
    (A) By blood relations
    (B) By how children are raised
    (C) By formal marriages
    (D) By support of one another

7. Describe the stages of human growth and development

True or False

1. _F_ A child takes three years from birth to be able to move around, communicate basic needs, and feed himself.

2. _F_ Physical development in infancy moves from the hands up to the head.

3. _T_ Tantrums are common among toddlers.

4. _F_ Preschool children are too young to know right from wrong.

5. _T_ Children learn to speak between the ages of 3 and 6.

6. _F_ From the ages of 6 to 10, children learn to get along with each other.

7. _T_ School-age children (6 to 10 years) develop cognitively and socially.

8. _T_ Preadolescents are often easy to get along with and are able to handle more responsibility than they were before.

9. _T_ Puberty is the stage of growth when secondary sex characteristics, such as body hair, appear.

10. _F_ Most adolescents do not feel that peer acceptance is important.

11. _T_ Adolescents may be moody due to changing hormones and body image concerns.

12. _F_ By 19 years of age, most young adults have stopped developing physically, psychologically, and socially.

13. _T_ One developmental task that most young adults undertake is to choose an occupation or career.

14. _F_ Middle-aged adults usually do not experience any physical changes due to aging.

15. _T_ By the time a person reaches late adulthood, he must adjust to the effects of aging.

16. _T_ Older adults have different capabilities depending upon their health.

17. _F_ As people age, they often become lonely, forgetful, and slow.

18. _F_ Diseases and illness are not a normal part of aging.

19. _T_ Many older adults can lead active and healthy lives.

20. _T_ Prejudice against older people is as unfair as prejudice against racial, ethnic, or religious groups.

21. _F_ Television and movies often present an accurate image of what it is like to grow old.

22. _T_ Skin becomes drier and less elastic with age.

23. _F_ Responses and reflexes quicken as a person ages.

24. _F_ Appetite increases with age.

25. _F_ Urinary elimination becomes less frequent in older adults.

26. _I_ Weakened immunity is a normal part of aging.

27. _F_ Depression is normal in the elderly.

28. _I_ The loss of ability to think logically is not a normal change of aging.

8. Discuss developmental disabilities

Short Answer

1. List three abilities that may be affected by developmental disabilities.

   • Mobility

   • self care

   • language

   _____

   _____

   _____

   _____

   _____

2. List four guidelines for caring for a resident who has an intellectual disability.

   • treat like an adult

   • be patient

   • encourage socializing

   • divide tasks into parts

   _____

   _____

   _____

   _____

   _____

   _____

9. Describe some types of mental health disorders

Multiple Choice

1. Uneasiness, worry, or fear, often about a situation or condition, is called
   (A) Anxiety
   (B) Withdrawal
   (C) Fatigue
   (D) Apathy

2. An intense, irrational fear of an object, place, or situation is called a
   (A) Depressive episode
   (B) Delusion
   (C) Phobia
   (D) Hallucination

3. Which of the following means a lack of interest in activities?
   (A) Guilt
   (B) Depression
   (C) Apathy
   (D) Delusion

4. A false sensory perception, such as a person seeing her mother who has been dead for many years in front of her, is a
   (A) Hallucination
   (B) Delusion
   (C) Phobia
   (D) Defense mechanism

5. A persistent false belief, such as a person believing that someone is controlling his thoughts, is a
   (A) Hallucination
   (B) Delusion
   (C) Phobia
   (D) Defense mechanism

6. Which of the following mental health disorders is characterized by changing moods, high energy, and big speeches?
   (A) Bipolar disorder
   (B) Panic disorder
   (C) Schizophrenia
   (D) Major depressive disorder

7. A method of treating mental health disorders that involves talking about one's problems with mental health professionals is called
    (A) Homeopathy
    (B) Psychotherapy
    (C) Electroconvulsive therapy
    (D) Massage therapy

10. Explain how to care for residents who are dying

Multiple Choice
Read each scenario below and choose which stage of grief the person is experiencing.

1. Mr. Cane was told two years ago that a tumor in his brain was inoperable and would eventually be fatal. Since that time, he has visited many specialists. Despite receiving the same diagnosis from every doctor, he continues to seek further opinions, insisting that each doctor try to remove the tumor.
    (A) Denial
    (B) Anger
    (C) Bargaining
    (D) Depression
    (E) Acceptance

2. Mrs. Tyler is dying of heart disease. One day as her nursing assistant, Annie, is assisting her with personal care, Mrs. Tyler lashes out at her. She tells Annie that she is a dumb girl who is wasting her life and does not deserve the many years she has left to live.
    (A) Denial
    (B) Anger
    (C) Bargaining
    (D) Depression
    (E) Acceptance

3. Mr. Lopez is dying of AIDS. He has called all of his friends to say goodbye and has discussed at length with his family the kind of memorial service he would like them to arrange.
    (A) Denial
    (B) Anger
    (C) Bargaining
    (D) Depression
    (E) Acceptance

4. Ms. Corke has always been lively and happy. Since she learning that she has Lou Gehrig's disease, however, her mood has changed drastically. Although she is still healthy enough to do activities, she rarely leaves her room or even changes out of her nightclothes.
    (A) Denial
    (B) Anger
    (C) Bargaining
    (D) Depression
    (E) Acceptance

5. Mr. Celasco has had lung cancer for several years. During that time, he has tried to quit smoking but has been unsuccessful. When he finds out that there are no further treatments for him to try, he pledges that he will give up smoking in exchange for a few more years of life.
    (A) Denial
    (B) Anger
    (C) Bargaining
    (D) Depression
    (E) Acceptance

Multiple Choice
Circle the letter of the answer that best completes the statement or answers the question.

6. Which of the following is a type of advance directive that appoints someone to make medical decisions for a person in the event he or she becomes unable to do so?
    (A) Advance decision
    (B) Living will
    (C) Durable power of attorney for health care
    (D) Do-not-resuscitate (DNR) order

7. A type of advance directive that outlines the medical care a person wants, or does not want, in case she becomes unable to make those decisions is called a
    (A) Safety data sheet
    (B) Living will
    (C) Do-not-resuscitate (DNR) order
    (D) Financial proxy

8. When medical personnel are instructed not to perform CPR if a person's breathing or heartbeat stops, it is referred to as a
   (A) Will
   (B) Power of attorney
   (C) Executor agreement
   (D) Do-not-resuscitate (DNR) order

Fill in the Blank

9. Nursing assistants should _bathe_ perspiring residents often; skin should be clean and dry.

10. Residents may not be able to communicate that they are in _pain_. NAs should observe for signs and report them.

11. Changes of position, back massage, skin care, mouth care, and proper body _alignment_ may help relieve pain.

12. _listening_ may be one of the most important things an NA can do for a resident who is dying. He should pay attention to these conversations.

13. _touch_ can be very important. Holding a dying resident's hand can be comforting.

14. The NA should not _avoid_ the dying person or his family and should not deny that death is approaching.

15. _hearing_ is usually the last sense to leave the body.

16. The NA should give _privacy_ for visits from clergy, family, and friends.

17. NAs should not discuss their personal _religious_ or spiritual beliefs with residents or their families or make recommendations.

Short Answer

18. List three legal rights to remember when working with residents who are dying.

• right to maintain hopefulness
• right to not die alone
• right to have questions answered honestly

19. Look at *The Dying Person's Bill of Rights* on pages 74–75 of the textbook. Pick two rights that you feel would be most important to you personally. Briefly describe why they are important to you.

• have questions answered honestly - I think ppl should know the truth about their health, even if it is unpleasant

• be free from pain - I think people that are dying should be made as comfortable as possible

Multiple Choice

20. After death, the muscles in the body become
    (A) Warm and pulsating
    (B) Bendable
    (C) Stiff and rigid
    (D) Hot and sharp

21. Caring for a body after death is called
    (A) Postmortem care
    (B) Mortician care
    (C) Funeral home care
    (D) Before-burial care

22. After death, the NA should place drainage pads under the body. These pads are most often needed under the
    (A) Arms
    (B) Perineum
    (C) Axillary area
    (D) Feet

23. If family members would like to remain with their loved one's body after death, the NA should
    (A) Let them do so
    (B) Inform them that the NA needs to ask the doctor first
    (C) Ask them to perform the postmortem care since they are staying with the body
    (D) Talk to them about the importance of organ donation

11. Define the goals of a hospice program

Multiple Choice

1. Hospice care is the term for compassionate care given to
    (A) Residents who have respiratory diseases
    (B) Residents who are dying
    (C) Residents with Parkinson's disease
    (D) Residents with developmental disabilities

2. Hospice care encourages residents to
    (A) Allow hospice care teams to handle all care decisions
    (B) Allow lawyers to make care decisions
    (C) Allow doctors to make care decisions
    (D) Participate in their own care as much as possible

3. Hospice goals focus on
    (A) Recovery of the dying person
    (B) Comfort and dignity of the dying person
    (C) Curing disease
    (D) Creating a will and other legal documents for the dying person

4. Focusing on pain relief, comfort, and managing symptoms is called _____ care.
    (A) Palliative
    (B) Personal
    (C) Professional
    (D) Pediatric

Short Answer

5. How do the goals of hospice care differ from those of long-term care?

    long-term goal is
    recovery, hospice
    goals are comfort +
    dignity.

    _____

    _____

    _____

    _____

Name: _____

4

Body Systems and Related Conditions

1. Describe the integumentary system

Fill in the Blank

1. The largest organ and system in the body is the _____skin_____.

2. Skin prevents _____injury_____ to internal organs.

3. Skin also prevents the loss of too much _____water_____, which is essential to life.

4. The skin is also a _____sense_____ organ that feels heat, cold, pain, touch, and pressure.

5. Blood vessels _____dilate_____, or widen, when the outside temperature is too high.

6. Blood vessels _____constrict_____, or narrow, when the outside temperature is too cold.

Normal or Sign/Symptom

Determine which of the following is a normal part of the aging process and which is a sign or symptom that needs to be reported to the nurse. Write an N for normal aging or an S for a sign/symptom to report.

7. _N_ Thinning skin

8. _S_ Bruises

9. _S_ Wounds

10. _N_ Wrinkles

11. _N_ Brown spots

12. _N_ Thinning of fatty tissue

13. _S_ Flaking skin

14. _N_ Thinning hair

15. _N_ Less elastic skin

16. _S_ Reddened skin

17. _S_ Swelling

18. _N_ Gray hair

19. _S_ Broken skin between the toes

Short Answer

Read the following paragraph and decide which items should be reported to the nurse.

20. A nursing assistant (NA) is providing care for a resident. As the NA is helping the resident turn over, she notices that the resident has a red spot above her buttocks and a bruise on her upper arm.

    the red spot and bruise should both be reported

2. Describe the musculoskeletal system and related conditions

True or False

1. _T_ The body is shaped by muscles, bones, ligaments, tendons, and cartilage.

2. _F_ The human body has 215 bones.   —206

3. _T_ Bones protect the body's organs.

4. _T_ Two bones meet at a joint.

5. __T__ Muscles allow movement of body parts.

6. __T__ Range of motion exercises help prevent problems related to immobility.

7. __T__ Atrophy occurs when a muscle weakens, decreases in size, and wastes away.

8. __T__ One way to prevent falls is to keep walkers or canes within reach.

Normal or Sign/Symptom

9. __S__ Bruising

10. __N__ Weakening of muscles

11. __N__ Loss of muscle tone

12. __S__ Change in ability to do routine movements

13. __N__ Loss of bone density

14. __N__ Increased brittleness of bones

15. __S__ Aches and pains

16. __N__ Loss of height

17. __S__ Pain during movement

18. __S__ Increased swelling of joints

19. __S__ White, shiny, or warm area over a joint

20. __N__ Slowing of body movement

Multiple Choice

21. Arthritis is a general term referring to _____ of the joints.
(A) Immobility
(B) Swelling
(C) Redness
(D) Stiffness

22. What happens to the body when a person suffers from an autoimmune illness?
(A) The circulatory system stops working, and blood backs up into the heart.
(B) The immune system attacks diseased tissue in the body.
(C) The immune system attacks normal tissue in the body.
(D) The musculoskeletal system becomes diseased.

23. Osteoarthritis is common in
(A) The elderly
(B) Infants
(C) Teenagers
(D) Nursing assistants

24. If an NA sees *NWB* on a resident's care plan, the resident
(A) Can support 100 percent of his body weight on one leg
(B) Can support some weight, but not all, on one or both legs
(C) Is unable to support any weight on one or both legs
(D) Can use stairs without assistance

25. Which side should a resident recovering from a hip replacement dress first?
(A) Affected (weaker) side
(B) Right side
(C) Unaffected (stronger) side
(D) Left side

26. Fractures are broken bones and are often caused by
(A) A high-fat diet
(B) Hypertension
(C) Osteoporosis
(D) Angina

27. What kind of pillow immobilizes and positions the hips and lower extremities after a hip replacement?
(A) An abduction pillow
(B) A body pillow
(C) A rotation pillow
(D) An extension pillow

28. Which of the following statements is true of a knee replacement?
(A) Blood clots are not normally a concern after a knee replacement.
(B) The person will not be able to bear weight on the knee again after a knee replacement.
(C) A knee replacement can help restore motion to the knee.
(D) Fluid intake should be restricted after a knee replacement.

Short Answer

Read the following paragraph and decide which items should be reported to the nurse.

29. A resident moves slowly as an NA helps him out of bed. The resident is not able to walk as far as he walked yesterday. The resident limps a little and occasionally makes a noise.

That the resident cannot walk as far as yesterday, limps, + makes noise should be reported.

3. Describe the nervous system and related conditions

Multiple Choice

1. The nervous system
   (A) Gives the body shape and structure
   (B) Controls and coordinates body function
   (C) Is the largest organ in the body
   (D) Pumps blood through the blood vessels to the cells

2. The two main parts of the nervous system are
   (A) The cardiovascular system and integumentary system
   (B) Neurons and receptors
   (C) The body and the brain
   (D) The central nervous system and peripheral nervous system

Normal or Sign/Symptom

3. _S_ Inability to move one side of the body
4. _S_ Depression
5. _S_ Fatigue with movement
6. _S_ Shaking

7. _S_ Decreased sense of heat and cold
8. _S_ Slurred speech
9. _S_ Decreased ability to perform ADLs
10. _N_ Slower reflexes
11. _S_ Trouble swallowing
12. _S_ Confusion
13. _S_ Decreased sensitivity of nerve endings in skin
14. _S_ Violent behavior
15. _S_ Minor short-term memory loss
16. _S_ Changes in vision

True or False

17. _F_ A resident who has paralysis after a stroke will usually not need physical therapy.
18. _T_ Leg exercises help improve circulation.
19. _F_ When helping with transfers or ambulation, the NA should stand on the resident's stronger side.
20. _T_ The NA should always use a gait belt for safety when helping a resident who has had a stroke to walk.
21. _F_ The NA should refer to the side that has been affected by the stroke as the "bad side" so that the resident will understand which side the NA is talking about.
22. _T_ Gestures and smiles are important when communicating with a resident who has had a stroke.
23. _T_ A resident who suffers confusion or memory loss due to a stroke may feel more secure if the NA keeps a routine of care.
24. _T_ A resident who has a loss of sensation could easily burn himself.
25. _T_ The NA should ask questions that can be answered with a "yes" or "no" when communicating with a resident who has had a stroke.

Name: _____

26. _F_   When assisting with dressing a resident who has had a stroke, the NA should dress the stronger side first.

Short Answer

Read each of the following statements and answer the questions.

27. Kate, a nursing assistant, is getting ready to take Mr. Elliot, who is recovering from a stroke, on a walk. Mr. Elliot has difficulty communicating and suffers from confusion. "Let's see," Kate says. "We can walk to the gardens, the activity room, or the front area. Now, where would you like to go?" What is wrong with the way Kate is communicating with Mr. Elliot?

She should ask
"yes" + "no"
questions

_____
_____
_____
_____
_____
_____

28. Kate notices that Mr. Elliot seems to be having trouble saying words clearly. He is beginning to get frustrated because he cannot tell Kate what he wants. Kate decides to ask only yes or no questions. She tells Mr. Elliot, "If you find it too difficult to speak right now, why don't you try nodding your head for yes and shaking your head for no." What is Kate doing right?

' asking yes + no
    questions
' being patient
_____
_____

_____
_____
_____
_____
_____
_____

True or False

29. _T_   Parkinson's disease is a progressive disease that causes a section of the brain to degenerate.

30. _T_   Parkinson's disease causes a shuffling gait and a mask-like facial expression.

31. _F_   Pill-rolling is something that people with Parkinson's disease must do before taking their medication.

32. _F_   A resident with Parkinson's disease should be discouraged from performing her own care to save energy.

Fill in the Blank

33. Multiple sclerosis causes the protective _myelin sheath_ for the nerves, spinal cord, and white matter of the brain to break down over time.

34. For a person with MS, nerves cannot send _messages_ to and from the brain in a normal way.

35. Symptoms of MS include _blurred_ vision, fatigue, tremors, poor balance, and trouble walking.

36. The NA should offer _rest_ periods as necessary for residents with MS.

37. The NA should give residents plenty of time to _respond_ because people with MS often have trouble forming their thoughts.

38. _Stress_ can worsen the effects of MS, so the NA should remain calm and listen to residents when they want to talk.

True or False

39. __T__ The effects of a spinal cord injury depend on the location of the injury and the force of impact.

40. __F__ The lower the injury on the spinal cord, the greater the loss of function will be.

41. __F__ Quadriplegia is a loss of function of the lower body and legs.

42. __F__ Rehabilitation is of little help for people who have had spinal cord injuries.

43. __T__ A resident with a head or spinal cord injury will need emotional support as well as physical help.

44. __T__ A resident with a spinal cord injury may not feel a burn because of a loss of sensation.

45. __T__ The NA should help the resident change positions at least every two hours to prevent pressure injuries.

46. __F__ A resident with a spinal cord injury should drink very little fluid to prevent urinary tract infection.

Short Answer

47. List the five sense organs of the body.

ears, eyes, nose tongue, skin

_____

_____

_____

Short Answer

Read the following paragraph and decide which items should be reported to the nurse.

48. An NA is assisting a resident with eating. It takes the resident a few seconds to take the napkin the NA is offering her. While the resident is eating, the NA notices she coughs while swallowing. The resident suddenly says that she cannot see the food on the left side of her plate.

• Coughing while swallowing

• Can't see food

_____

_____

_____

_____

_____

_____

_____

_____

_____

4. Describe the circulatory system and related conditions

Fill in the Blank

1. The circulatory system is made up of the ___heart___, blood, and blood ___vessels___.

2. The blood carries food, ___oxygen___, and other substances cells need to function.

3. The circulatory system removes ___waste___ products from cells.

Normal or Sign/Symptom

4. __S__ Severe headache

5. __S__ Heart pumps less efficiently

6. __S__ Chest pain

7. __S__ Swelling of hands or feet

8. __S__ Changes in pulse rate

9. __S__ Bluish hands or feet

10. __N__ Fatigue

11. __S__ Shortness of breath

Short Answer

12. What is the consistent blood pressure measurement at which a person is diagnosed with hypertension?

    _____ 130/80 _____

13. What are three possible causes of hypertension?

    • atherosclerosis

    • kidney disease

    • pregnancy

Coronary Artery Disease (CAD)

True or False

14. __T__ Coronary artery disease (CAD) lowers the supply of blood, oxygen, and nutrients to the heart and can lead to heart attack or stroke.

15. __F__ The heart needs more oxygen when the body is at rest.

16. __T__ The pain of angina pectoris is usually described as pressure or tightness in the left side of the chest.

17. __T__ A person suffering from angina pectoris may sweat, look pale, and have trouble breathing.

18. __T__ If a person with CAD rests, it helps the blood flow return to normal.

19. __F__ A nursing assistant can administer nitroglycerin to a resident when the resident requests it.

20. __T__ A residents who has CAD may need to avoid heavy meals and intense exercise.

Short Answer

21. List six things that may be included in a cardiac rehabilitation program.

    • exercise

    • special diet

    • Medication

    • Stop Smoking

    • regular blood testing

    • avoid heavy meals

Congestive Heart Failure (CHF)

Fill in the Blank

22. Congestive heart failure can be treated and controlled with

    ___ medications ___.

23. Medications help remove excess

    ___ fluid ___.

    This means more trips to the

    ___ bathroom ___.

24. Limited ___ sodium ___

    or ___ fluid restrictions ___

    may be prescribed.

25. Residents may need to be

    ___ weighed ___ at the same time

    every day.

26. Extra ___ pillows ___

    may help residents who have trouble breathing.

27. A common side effect of CHF medication is

    ___ dizziness ___.

Multiple Choice

28. Peripheral vascular disease (PVD) is a condition in which the legs, feet, arms, or hands do not have enough
    (A Flexibility
    (B) Fat
    (C) Blood circulation
    (D) Fluids

29. PVD is caused by
    (A) Weakened bones
    (B) Weakened heart muscle due to damage
    (C) Infection of the arteries
    (D) Fatty deposits in blood vessels

Short Answer

Read the following paragraph and decide which items should be reported to the nurse.

30. An NA is giving a resident a bed bath. The NA notices that the resident's fingertips are blue and her feet are swollen. The resident complains of being tired.

    • blue finger tips
    • Swollen feet
    • complaints of being tired

5. Describe the respiratory system and related conditions

True or False

1. __T__ Respiration occurs in the lungs.

2. __F__ Expiration is breathing in.

3. __T__ The respiratory system brings oxygen into the body and removes carbon dioxide.

4. __T__ Regular exercise and movement should be encouraged.

Normal or Sign/Symptom

5. __S__ Decreased lung strength and capacity

6. __S__ Discolored sputum

7. __S__ Need to sit after mild exertion

8. __S__ Shallow breathing

9. __S__ Bluish legs

10. __S__ Weaker voice

11. __S__ Coughing

12. __N__ Nasal congestion

13. __S__ Change in respiratory rate

Multiple Choice

14. Residents with chronic obstructive pulmonary disease (COPD) have difficulty with
    (A) Breathing
    (B) Urination
    (C) Losing weight
    (D) Vision

15. For a person with COPD, a common fear is
    (A) Constipation
    (B) Incontinence
    (C) Not being able to breathe
    (D) Heart attack

16. What is the best position for a resident with COPD?
    (A) Lying flat on his back
    (B) Sitting upright
    (C) Lying on his stomach
    (D) Lying on his side

17. Part of the NA's role in caring for a resident with COPD includes
    (A) Being calm and supportive
    (B) Adjusting oxygen levels
    (C) Making changes in the resident's diet
    (D) Doing everything for the resident as much as possible

18. Chronic bronchitis and emphysema are grouped under
    (A) Chronic obstructive pulmonary disease, or COPD
    (B) Muscular dystrophy, or MD
    (C) Hypertension, or HTN
    (D) Coronary artery disease, or CAD

Short Answer

Read the following paragraph and decide which items should be reported to the nurse.

19. While the NA is providing care, a resident makes a wheezing sound when he breathes. After turning over in bed, the resident says he needs to rest before continuing. He begins to cough.

- wheezing
- coughing

6. Describe the urinary system and related conditions

Short Answer

1. List the two vital functions of the urinary system.

- eliminates waste
- maintains water balance

2. What is one reason why the female bladder is more likely to become infected with bacteria than the male bladder?

- shorter urethra
- closer to anus

Normal or Sign/Symptom

3. _S_ Pain during urination

4. _S_ Bladder does not empty completely

5. _S_ Bladder feels full or painful

6. _S_ Pain in kidney region

7. _S_ Changes in color of urine

8. _S_ Urinary incontinence

9. _S_ Inadequate fluid intake

True or False

10. _T_ To avoid infection, women should wipe the perineal area from front to back after elimination.

11. _F_ Limiting fluid intake helps prevent urinary tract infections (UTIs).

12. _F_ Taking baths, rather than showers, helps prevent UTIs.

Short Answer

Read the following paragraph and decide which items should be reported to the nurse.

13. An NA always needs to give a resident a urinal before and after helping him walk. Today the NA notices that the resident's urine is cloudy and has a strong odor. When the NA visits the resident later, she sees urine on his bed linens.

- Cloudy, odorous urine
- urine on bed linens

7. Describe the gastrointestinal system and related conditions

Short Answer

1. Explain three functions of the gastrointestinal system.

   - digestion
   - absorbtion
   - elimination
   _____
   _____
   _____
   _____

Normal or Sign/Symptom

2. _N_ Flatulence
3. _S_ Decreased saliva
4. _N_ Dulled sense of taste
5. _S_ Black stool
6. _S_ Fecal incontinence
7. _N_ Decreased absorption of nutrients
8. _S_ Diarrhea
9. _N_ Less efficient digestion
10. _S_ Heartburn

Crossword

Across

15. Keeping the body in this position during sleep may help symptoms of gastroesophageal reflux disease

16. Enlarged veins in the rectum that cause itching and burning

Down

11. Treatment of constipation often includes eating more of this

12. An artificial opening in the body

13. The frequent elimination of liquid or semi-liquid feces

14. Abbreviation for gastroesophageal reflux disease

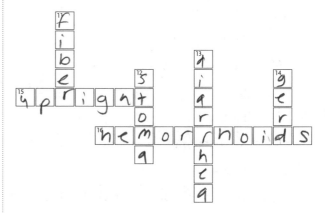

Short Answer

Read the following paragraph and decide which items should be reported to the nurse.

17. Mr. Sanchez is not eating as much as he used to. He has lost two pounds since the NA last weighed him. He says he just is not as hungry lately.

   - not eating as much
   - weight loss
   - loss of apetite
   _____
   _____
   _____
   _____

8. Describe the endocrine system and related conditions

Fill in the Blank

1. The endocrine system is made up of _glands_.

2. _hormones_ are chemical substances created by the body that control numerous body functions.

3. As a person ages, the body is less able to handle _stress_.

Normal or Sign/Symptom

4. _S_ Excessive perspiration

5. _S_ Dizziness

6. _S_ Hyperactivity

7. _S_ Blurred vision

8. _N_ Less able to handle stress

9. _S_ Irritability

10. _S_ Headache

11. _N_ Reduced insulin production

12. _S_ Hunger

13. _N_ Decrease in progesterone levels

14. _S_ Confusion

15. _S_ Weakness

Multiple Choice

16. Diabetes is a condition in which the pancreas does not produce enough or properly use
(A) Insulin
(B) Glucose
(C) Growth hormones
(D) Adrenaline

17. Sugars collecting in the blood cause problems with
(A) Breathing
(B) Circulation
(C) Pain level
(D) Ambulation

18. Type 1 diabetes
(A) Continues throughout a person's life
(B) Is most common in the elderly
(C) Is first treated with surgery
(D) Does not require a change of diet

19. Changes in the circulatory system from diabetes can cause
(A) Hair loss
(B) Heart attack and stroke
(C) Multiple sclerosis
(D) COPD

20. The most common form of diabetes is
(A) Pre-diabetes
(B) Gestational diabetes
(C) Type 1 diabetes
(D) Type 2 diabetes

21. Poor circulation and impaired wound healing may result in
(A) Urinary tract infections
(B) Cancer
(C) Leg and foot ulcers
(D) An autoimmune disease

22. Gangrene can lead to
(A) Loss of bowel control
(B) Peripheral vascular disease
(C) Congestive heart failure
(D) Amputation

23. What condition occurs when a person's blood glucose level is above normal but not high enough for a diagnosis of type 2 diabetes?
(A) Gestational diabetes
(B) Type 1 diabetes
(C) Pre-diabetes
(D) Hyperglycemia

24. Careful _____ care is vitally important for people with diabetes.
(A) Foot
(B) Hair
(C) Facial
(D) Mouth

Short Answer
Read the following paragraph and decide which items should be reported to the nurse.

25. An NA walks into a resident's room and notices that the resident has just finished drinking a glass of water. The resident asks the NA to refill her water pitcher because it is empty. The NA had just filled it 15 minutes ago. When the NA returns with the pitcher, she sees that the resident is sweating even though the room feels cool.

• increase in water intake
• sweating in cool room

_____
_____
_____
_____
_____
_____
_____
_____
_____
_____

9. Describe the reproductive system and related conditions

Multiple Choice

1. The reproductive system allows humans to
   (A) Move and speak
   (B) Create human life
   (C) Think logically
   (D) Fight disease

2. The male and female sex glands are called the
   (A) Adrenals
   (B) Ureters
   (C) Gonads
   (D) Urethras

3. The end of menstrual periods in females is called
   (A) Degeneration
   (B) Discontinuation
   (C) Menopause
   (D) Suspension

Normal or Sign/Symptom

4. _S_ Erectile dysfunction (male)

5. _N_ Decrease in estrogen (female)

6. _S_ Swelling of genitals

7. _N_ Enlarged prostate gland (male)

8. _N_ End of menstruation (female)

9. _S_ Discharge from penis or vagina

10. _S_ Blood in stool

11. _S_ Painful intercourse

12. _N_ Decrease in sperm production (male)

13. _S_ Sores on genitals

14. _S_ Discomfort with urination

15. _S_ Itchy genitals

True or False

16. _F_ Benign prostatic hypertrophy is a fairly common disorder that occurs in both women and men as they age.

17. _T_ Vaginitis can be caused by bacteria, protozoa, or fungi.

Short Answer

Read the following paragraph and decide which items should be reported to the nurse.

18. An NA notices that a resident has trouble urinating, and his face indicates that he is in pain. The resident later tells the NA that he has a sore area on his penis.

   - trouble urinating
   - looks to be in pain
   - Sore area on penis

   _____
   _____
   _____
   _____
   _____
   _____
   _____
   _____
   _____
   _____
   _____

10. Describe the immune and lymphatic systems and related conditions

Fill in the Blank

1. The immune system protects the body from disease-causing __bacteria__, viruses, and organisms.

2. __Nonspecific__ immunity protects the body from disease in general.

3. __Specific__ immunity protects against a disease that is invading the body at a given time.

4. The lymphatic system removes excess __fluids__ and waste products from the tissues.

5. __Lymph__ is a clear yellowish fluid that carries disease-fighting cells. The cells are called __lymphocytes__.

Normal or Sign/Symptom

6. __S__ Swelling of lymph nodes

7. __S__ Increased fatigue

8. __N__ Decreased response to vaccines

9. __N__ Increased risk of infection

Multiple Choice

10. Care for a person who has HIV or AIDS should focus on
    (A) Helping to find a cure for HIV
    (B) Preventing visits from friends and family so as not to infect them
    (C) Providing relief of symptoms and preventing infection
    (D) Letting the person know about new treatments and medications that are successful in treating the disease

11. If a resident with AIDS has a poor appetite, the nursing assistant should
    (A) Give the resident an over-the-counter appetite stimulant
    (B) Serve familiar and favorite foods
    (C) Let the resident know that if he does not eat, he might die
    (D) Discuss this with the resident's friends to see what they recommend doing

12. Residents who have AIDS and have infections of the mouth may need to eat food that is
    (A) Spicy
    (B) Low in acid
    (C) Dry
    (D) Very hot

13. A resident with AIDS who is nauseated and vomiting should
    (A) Eat mostly dairy products
    (B) Eat high-fat foods
    (C) Drink liquids
    (D) Reduce liquid intake

14. Fluids are important for residents who have diarrhea because
    (A) Diarrhea rapidly depletes the body of fluids
    (B) Diarrhea can be prevented by drinking a lot of fluids
    (C) Diarrhea is an infection that can be flushed out by fluids
    (D) Diarrhea can make a resident's throat dry

15. The following is helpful in dealing with numbness, tingling, and pain in the feet:
    (A) Wrapping feet in elastic bandages
    (B) Wearing narrow, closed shoes
    (C) Using a bed cradle
    (D) Tucking in bed sheets tightly

16. If a resident with cancer is experiencing pain, the NA should
    (A) Assist with comfort measures
    (B) Let the resident know that there is little the NA can do
    (C) Suggest types of pain medication the resident can take
    (D) Give the resident an injection of pain medication

17. Which of the following would be the best response from the NA if a resident with cancer expresses fear about her condition?
    (A) "I know exactly what you're going through because my mother had the same condition."
    (B) "I've read about a new medication that helps cancer like yours."
    (C) "You'll be feeling better in no time."
    (D) "I understand you're scared. Do you feel like talking?"

18. To help promote proper nutrition for a resident with cancer, the NA should do the following:
    (A) Use metal utensils when serving meals
    (B) Serve favorite foods that are nutritious
    (C) Restrict nutritional supplements
    (D) Serve foods with little nutritional content

Short Answer
Read the following paragraph and decide which items should be reported to the nurse.

19. Ms. Gallagher is running a fever. She complains of being tired and mentions that she has had three bouts of diarrhea in the last hour.

    • fever
    • fatigue
    • diarrhea
    _____
    _____
    _____
    _____
    _____

Body Systems and Related Conditions

5

Confusion, Dementia, and Alzheimer's Disease

1. Discuss confusion and delirium

Short Answer

1. What are ten actions that a nursing assistant can take when helping care for a resident who is confused?

    • dont leave them alone

    • speak in low tone of voice

    • introduce each time you see them

    • be patient

    • remind them of their name, date, + location

    • talk about plans for the day/keep a routine

    • promote selfcare, independence

    • report observations

    • encourage use of eyeglasses + hearing aids

    • explain what you're doing simple instructions

2. Name four possible causes of delirium.

    • infections

    • disease

    • fluid imbalances

    • poor nutrition

2. Describe dementia and discuss Alzheimer's disease

True or False

1. __T__ Dementia is the loss of mental abilities such as thinking, remembering, reasoning, and communicating.

2. __F__ Dementia is something that happens as every person gets older.

3. __T__ Alzheimer's disease is the most common cause of dementia in the elderly.

4. __F__ Men are more likely to have Alzheimer's disease than women.

5. __T__ Alzheimer's disease causes tangled nerve fibers and protein deposits to form in the brain, eventually causing dementia.

6. __T__ There is no cure for Alzheimer's disease.

7. __F__ There is one simple exam that is performed to diagnose Alzheimer's disease.

8. __T__ Each person with Alzheimer's disease will show different signs at different times.

9. __T__ Most Alzheimer's disease victims will eventually need constant care.

10. __F__ Symptoms of Alzheimer's disease typically appear suddenly.

3. List strategies for better communication with residents with Alzheimer's disease

Scenarios

Read each scenario below and state an appropriate response.

1. Mrs. Hays, a resident with Alzheimer's disease (AD), has awakened from her nap and does not recognize her room or anyone around her.

   Smile, speak clearly and reasuringly, introduce yourself + remind them of name, date, + location.

2. Kena, a nursing assistant (NA), has been trying to give Mr. Collins, a resident with AD, a bath. Mr. Collins has become agitated and is asking Kena "Who are you?" over and over again, although Kena has already identified herself twice.

   continue to intro introduce herself, repeat directions, + reschedule bath for when they are less agitated.

3. Mrs. Hays has been telling Kena a story about her niece. She is showing Kena a necklace that her niece gave her as a gift. She is having trouble remembering the word *necklace* and is getting upset.

   encourage them to gsture, or find another word that may sound familiar, comfort them w/ touch or a hug

4. Kena is helping Mr. Collins get ready to go to dinner. Kena asks him to put on his shoes, but Mr. Collins does not understand what Kena wants him to do.

   break the activity into simple steps + encourage them to do what they can.

Multiple Choice

5. When communicating with a resident with AD, the nursing assistant should
   (A) Quietly approach the resident from behind
   (B) Stand as close as possible to the resident
   (C) Communicate in a loud, busy place to help cheer up the resident
   (D) Speak slowly, using a lower tone of voice than normal

6. If a resident is frightened or anxious, which of the following should the NA do?
   (A) Check his body language so he does not appear tense or hurried
   (B) Turn up the television to try to distract the resident
   (C) Use complex, longer sentences to calm the resident
   (D) Give multiple instructions at one time so that the resident has time to understand them

7. If a resident perseverates, this means he is
   (A) Repeating words, phrases, questions, or actions
   (B) Suggesting words that sound correct
   (C) Hallucinating or having delusions
   (D) Gesturing instead of speaking

8. If a resident does not remember how to perform basic tasks, the NA should
   (A) Do everything for him
   (B) Encourage the resident to do what he can
   (C) Skip explaining each activity
   (D) Say "don't" as often as the NA feels is necessary

4. List and describe interventions for problems with common activities of daily living (ADLs)

Short Answer

For each of the following statements, write good idea *if the statement is a good idea for residents with Alzheimer's disease or* bad idea *if the statement is a bad idea.*

1. Use nonslip mats, tub seats, and handholds to ensure safety during bathing.
   good idea

2. Always bathe the resident at the same time every day, even if she is agitated.
   bad idea

3. Break tasks down into simple steps, explaining one step at a time.
   good idea

4. Do not attempt to groom the resident; most people with Alzheimer's disease do not care about their appearance.
   bad idea

5. Choose clothes that are simple to put on.
   good idea

6. If the resident is incontinent, do not give him fluids, because it makes the problem worse.
   bad idea

7. Mark the bathroom with a sign or picture as a reminder to use it and where it is.
   good idea

8. Check the skin regularly for signs of irritation.
   good idea

9. Follow Standard Precautions when caring for the resident.
   good idea

10. Do not encourage exercise, as this will make the resident more agitated.
    bad idea

11. Serve finger foods if the resident tends to wander during meals.
    good idea

12. Schedule meals at the same time every day.
    good idea

13. Serve new kinds of foods as often as possible to stimulate the resident.
    bad idea

14. Put only one kind of food on the plate at a time.
    bad idea

15. Use plain white dishes for serving food.
    good idea

16. Do not encourage independence, as this can lead to aggressive behavior.
    bad idea

17. Reward positive behavior with smiles and warm touches.
    good idea

5. List and describe interventions for common difficult behaviors related to Alzheimer's disease

Scenarios

For each description below, identify the behavior that the resident with Alzheimer's disease is exhibiting. Describe one way of dealing with it.

1. Mrs. Donne gets upset at about 9:00 p.m. every night. She repeatedly asks for snacks or drinks and refuses to go to bed.
   • Sundowning
   - provide snacks, a soothing activity or music, and make sure their bedtime is the same every day

2. Mr. Noble is playing chess with a friend and becomes angry when he loses the game. He shoves his friend, and when the NA approaches, he tells her he is going to hit her.

• Violent behavior
They should call for
help, step out of reach
+ stay calm, avoid
leaving them alone, +
try to remove triggers.

3. Mrs. Martin gets very upset every time she sees the president on television. She yells at the screen and tells everyone what a poor state our country is in.

• agitation
• remove the trigger +
avoid it in the future,
reduce noise/distractions,
stay calm + use a
low soothing voice.

4. Ms. Desmond used to enjoy talking to people and reading, but lately she does not seem to enjoy anything. She sleeps most of the day and never talks to anyone unless she is asked to.

• depression
- report signs to nurse,
encourage self-care +
activity, encourage
social interaction

5. Whenever Mr. Fejer does not like what is being served for dinner, he bangs on the table with his fists and shouts about how much he hates his food. When people try to get him to stop, he only grows louder.

- catastrophic reaction
- remove triggers + help
them focus on a
soothing activity

6. Ms. Storey is walking around the facility asking everyone she meets what time it is. Even though she has been told several times, she still seems unsatisfied and keeps asking the question.

- wandering
remove causes, let
them wander in a
safe space, redirect
their attention

7. About an hour before dinner every night, Ms. Foley starts walking up and down the hall as quickly as she can. She does not speak to or acknowledge anyone else while she is doing this.

- wandering
remove causes, let
her wander in a safe
space, redirect
attention

8. Whenever a female resident comes into the television room, Mr. Radcliffe tells her that he loves her and starts removing his clothes. If she stays in the room long enough, he will ask her to take off her clothes, too.

    - unappropriate sexual behavior
    Stay calm, distract the resident or direct them to a private area, report to nurse.

9. Mrs. Rowling loves the color red. She has a lot of red clothing that she enjoys wearing. Whenever she sees a piece of red clothing, even in another resident's room, she picks it up and takes it back to her room.

    - hoarding / rummaging
    - label all belongings w/ name + room #, regularly check areas where they store items

10. Mr. Bullis tells his NA that his wife has just called him. She is coming to pick him up, and they are going to dinner at the place they went on their first date. The NA knows that his wife has been dead for several years and their favorite restaurant has long since closed down.

    - hallucinations / delusions
    - not argue w/ them, ignore harmless delusions, reassure the resident

6. Describe creative therapies for residents with Alzheimer's disease

Scenarios

For each situation described below, identify the therapy that the nursing assistant is using.

1. Ms. Lee misses her husband, who has been dead for ten years, very much. Keisha, an NA who works with her, always asks about her life with her husband and what it was like. Ms. Lee seems to enjoy telling Keisha stories about what they did when they were young and how happy she was when they were together.

    Reminiscence therapy

2. Mr. Elking tells Keisha that he has a date with Rose, the pretty girl who lives across the street. He is going to take her dancing and out to a movie. Keisha knows that Rose lived in his neighborhood when he was a teenager and that he has not seen her for years. Keisha knows that Mr. Elking rarely gets out of bed. Instead of correcting him, Keisha asks him what kind of movie they are going to see and what he thinks he should wear.

    Validation therapy

3. Mr. Tennant sometimes gets depressed, especially in the evenings. Keisha knows that he loves classical music, so she starts playing it for him in the evenings a little before he usually starts feeling sad. He sorts through albums and places them in stacks.

    Music therapy

Name: _____

6

Personal Care Skills

1. Explain personal care of residents

True or False

1. ___T___ Promoting independence is part of how a nursing assistant (NA) cares for residents.

2. ___T___ Styling one's hair is part of grooming oneself.

3. ___F___ Perineal care is care of the fingernails and toenails.

4. ___F___ It is best for the NA to make the decisions about when and where procedures will be done.

5. ___T___ Having care explained before it is performed is a resident's legal right.

6. ___T___ The NA should knock and wait for permission to enter a resident's room.

7. ___T___ Personal care provides the NA with an opportunity to observe a resident's mental state.

8. ___F___ If a resident appears tired during a procedure, the NA should encourage him to keep going so that the procedure is more efficient.

9. ___F___ Before leaving a resident's room, the NA should leave the bed in its highest position.

10. ___F___ The call light should always be left where the NA can easily reach it when she returns to the room.

2. Identify guidelines for providing skin care and preventing pressure injuries

Crossword
Across

2. The bottom sheet on a resident's bed must be kept tight and free from w_____.

5. Cloth-covered items that keep the hand or fingers in a normal, natural position

6. A problem that can result from pulling a resident across the sheet when transferring him

8. Skin should be kept clean and _____.

Down

1. Keeps covers from resting on the legs and feet

3. One type of material that prevents air from circulating, causing the skin to sweat

4. At a minimum, the number of hours at which immobile residents should be repositioned

7. Skin this color should not be massaged

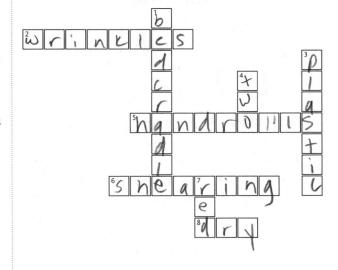

Personal Care Skills

Labeling

For each position shown, list the areas at risk for pressure injuries.

Lateral Position

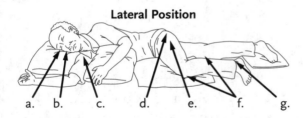

a. b. c. d. e. f. g.

9. Lateral Position
    a. side of head
    b. ear
    c. shoulder
    d. hip
    e. greater trochanter
    f. knees
    g. ankles

Prone Position

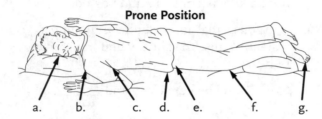

a. b. c. d. e. f. g.

10. Prone Position
    a. cheek
    b. collar bone
    c. breasts
    d. abdomen
    e. genitals
    f. knees
    g. toes

Supine Position

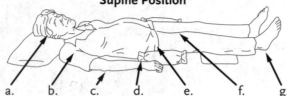

a. b. c. d. e. f. g.

11. Supine Position
    a. back of head
    b. shoulder blades
    c. elbows
    d. buttocks
    e. sacrum
    f. between legs
    g. heels

True or False

12. __T__ With a stage 1 pressure injury, skin is intact but may appear red and may be warmer than the area around it.

13. __F__ Immobile residents should be repositioned every four hours.

14. __T__ Areas of the body where bone is close to the skin are at a higher risk for skin breakdown.

15. __F__ Residents seated in wheelchairs do not need to be repositioned.

16. __F__ The NA should massage any red areas he notices.

17. __T__ Proper nutrition helps keep the skin healthy.

18. __F__ When transferring or positioning residents, the NA should pull them slowly across the sheets to make the job easier.

19. __T__ Another name for pressure injuries is decubitus ulcers.

20. __F__ Common sites for pressure injuries are the chest, nose, and hands.

21. __T__ A type of device that helps support and align a limb is called an orthosis.

Matching
Use each letter only once.

22. __B__ Bed cradle

23. __D__ Bony prominences

24. __C__ Draw sheet

25. __A__ Footboard

26. __E__ Handrolls

27. __G__ Orthotic device

28. __H__ Pressure points

29. __F__ Trochanter rolls

(A) Placed against the feet to keep them properly aligned and to prevent foot drop

(B) Keeps bed covers from resting on the legs

(C) Used to help residents who cannot help with turning or moving in bed; helps prevent skin damage from shearing

(D) Areas of the body where the bone lies close to the skin

(E) Keeps fingers in a natural position

(F) Rolled towels used to keep the hips and legs from turning outward

(G) Helps support and align a limb and improve its functioning

(H) Areas of the body that bear much of its weight

3. Describe guidelines for assisting with bathing

Multiple Choice

1. A partial bath includes washing a resident's
   (A) Feet
   (B) Genitals
   (C) Legs
   (D) Back

2. Which of the following should be used to wash the resident's face when giving a bed bath?
   (A) Washcloth and water
   (B) Washcloth and soap
   (C) Brush and soap
   (D) Washcloth and moisturizing cream

3. Who is best able to choose a comfortable water temperature for the resident?
   (A) The nursing assistant
   (B) The resident
   (C) The resident's family member
   (D) The nurse

4. How hot should the water be when shampooing a resident's hair?
   (A) No higher than 105°F
   (B) No higher than 110°F
   (C) No higher than 115°F
   (D) No higher than 120°F

5. The resident's perineum should be washed
   (A) Twice a day
   (B) Once a day
   (C) Once a week
   (D) Every other day

6. Which of the following products should be used when giving a shower or tub bath?
   (A) Baby powder
   (B) Body oil
   (C) Shampoo
   (D) Talcum powder

7. When should gloves be changed during a bed bath?
   (A) Before washing the perineal area
   (B) Before washing the arms and axillae
   (C) Before washing the hands
   (D) Before washing the face

4. Describe guidelines for assisting with grooming

Short Answer

1. List one benefit of regular grooming.

   - makes the resident feel good about how they look

2. Describe two grooming routines that are important in your life. Why do you think routines are important to people even when they are ill?

   • hair styling
   • nail care

   even when ppl are ill they want to feel like they look nice and grooming can also make them more comfortubly

Name: _____

_____
_____
_____
_____

3. Where on the foot should an NA not apply lotion when giving foot care?

    between the toes

4. Why should an NA wear gloves while shaving a resident?

    Shaving may
    cause bleeding

5. Why should electric razors not be used near any water or when oxygen is in use?

    may cause
    electrocution

6. The textbook states that when combing or brushing hair, the NA should "avoid childish hairstyles." Why do you think this statement is included?

    adults don't like
    to be treated like
    children : it's a
    matter of respect.

7. What are ways to prevent the spread of lice?

    • dont shave combs/
      brushes/wigs or hats
    • report signs of lice

5. List guidelines for assisting with dressing

Multiple Choice

1. Which of the following would be the best type of clothing for a resident to wear during the day?
    (A) A comfortable nightgown
    (B) A clean blouse and pair of pants
    (C) A flannel pajama top and bottoms
    (D) A bathrobe and slippers

2. For a resident who has weakness or paralysis on one side, the NA should place the _____ arm or leg through the garment first.
    (A) Stronger
    (B) Weaker
    (C) Right
    (D) Left

3. When undressing a resident who has weakness or paralysis on one side, the NA should start with the _____ side.
    (A) Stronger
    (B) Weaker
    (C) Right
    (D) Left

4. The resident's clothing for the day should be chosen by the
   (A) Resident
   (B) Resident's friend
   (C) Nursing assistant
   (D) Physical therapist

6. Identify guidelines for proper oral hygiene

Short Answer

1. How often should oral care be performed? When should it be done?

   · twice a day
   · after breakfast &
     dinner

2. List eight signs to observe and report about the mouth when performing oral care.

   · coated or swollen tongue
   · ulcers
   · flaky white spots
   · dry, cracked lips
   · loose, chipped, broken
     teeth
   · swollen, irritated, bleeding
     gums
   · breath that is bad or fruity
   · mouth pain

3. What is aspiration? How can the NA help prevent aspiration during oral care of unconscious residents?

   - inhalation of food, fluid,
     foreign material

   - use swabs soaked
     in tiny amounts of
     fluid

7. Explain guidelines for assisting with toileting

Multiple Choice

1. A fracture pan is used for voiding for
   (A) Any resident who cannot get out of bed
   (B) Residents who cannot raise their hips
   (C) Residents who have problems with urinary incontinence
   (D) Residents who have difficulty urinating

2. Men will generally use a _____ for urination when they cannot get out of bed.
   (A) Urinal
   (B) Fracture pan
   (C) Toilet
   (D) Portable commode

3. Residents who can get out of bed but cannot walk to the bathroom may use a(n)
   (A) Toilet
   (B) Urinal
   (C) Portable commode
   (D) Indwelling catheter

4. Another name for portable commode is
   (A) Toilet attachment
   (B) Portable urinal
   (C) Bedside commode
   (D) Hat

Name: _____

5. Which of the following statements is true?
(A) When handling body wastes, the NA should wear gloves.
(B) The NA should put the waste container on the overbed table when it is not in use.
(C) The NA should store elimination equipment on the resident's side table.
(D) Containers used for elimination should be cleaned after every two uses.

Short Answer

6. Why should the NA note the color, odor, and qualities of urine and stool after a resident uses a bedpan, urinal, or commode?

• provides nurse w/ information to assess resident

8. Explain the guidelines for safely positioning and moving residents

Labeling
Label each position that is illustrated below.

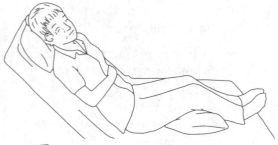

1. ____ Fowlers ____

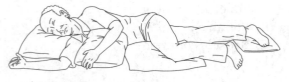

2. ____ Lateral ____

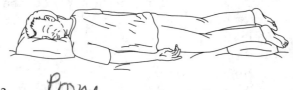

3. ____ Prone ____

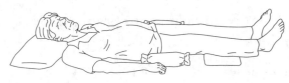

4. ____ Supine ____

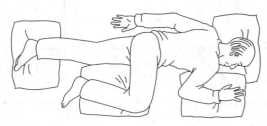

5. ____ Sims ____

Multiple Choice

6. Why do residents who spend a lot of time in bed or wheelchairs need to be repositioned often?
(A) Repositioning keeps sheets and cushions from getting dirty.
(B) They are at risk of skin breakdown and pressure injuries.
(C) Staff need to make sure residents are awakened regularly.
(D) Repositioning helps prevent boredom.

7. In this position, the resident is lying on either side:
(A) Supine
(B) Lateral
(C) Prone
(D) Fowler's

8. In this position, the resident is lying on his stomach:
(A) Sims'
(B) Lateral
(C) Prone
(D) Fowler's

9. Some residents have a side of the body that is weaker than the other one. The weaker side of the body should be referred to as the
   (A) Released side
   (B) Separated side
   (C) Ambulated side
   (D) Involved side

10. A draw sheet is used to
    (A) Make changing the bottom bedsheet easier
    (B) Help residents sleep better
    (C) Reposition residents without causing shearing
    (D) Prevent urinary incontinence

11. Logrolling is
    (A) A way to measure the weight of a resident who is bedbound
    (B) One way to record vital signs for residents who cannot get out of bed easily
    (C) Moving a resident as a unit without disturbing alignment
    (D) A special method of bedmaking

12. Dangling is
    (A) Lying in the supine position
    (B) Doing a few sit-ups in bed to get used to the upright position
    (C) Elevating the resident's feet with pillows
    (D) A way to help residents regain balance before standing up

13. A resident in the Fowler's position is
    (A) In a semi-sitting position
    (B) Lying flat on his back
    (C) In a left side-lying position
    (D) Lying on his stomach

14. Which of the following statements is true of working with residents in wheelchairs?
    (A) Before transferring a resident, the NA should make sure the wheelchair is unlocked and movable.
    (B) The NA should check the resident's alignment in the chair after a transfer is complete.
    (C) To fold a standard wheelchair, the NA should turn it upside-down to make the seat flatten.
    (D) All residents will need their NAs to transfer them to their wheelchairs.

15. The following piece of equipment may be used to help transfer residents who are unable to bear weight on their legs:
    (A) Sling
    (B) Slide board
    (C) Wheeled table
    (D) Folded blanket

16. Which of the following statements is true of mechanical, or hydraulic, lifts?
    (A) When doing this type of transfer, it is safer for one person to transfer the resident by himself.
    (B) The legs of the stand need to be closed, in their narrowest position, before helping the resident into the lift.
    (C) Lifts help prevent injury to the nursing assistant and the resident.
    (D) It is best to use mechanical lifts when moving residents a long distance.

17. When applying a transfer belt, the NA should place it
    (A) Around the wheelchair's backrest
    (B) Underneath the resident's clothing, on bare skin
    (C) Over the resident's clothing and around the waist
    (D) Around the NA's waist so the resident can hold on to it

18. If a resident starts to fall during the transfer, the NA's best response would be to
    (A) Bend her knees and lower the resident to the floor
    (B) Catch the resident under the arms to stop the fall
    (C) Move away and allow the resident to fall on her own
    (D) Have the resident fall on top of her to break the fall

Personal Care Skills

7

Basic Nursing Skills

1. Explain admission, transfer, and discharge of a resident

Fill in the Blank

1. _____admission_____ is often the first time a nursing assistant (NA) meets a new resident.

2. The NA should try to make sure the resident has a positive _____impression_____ of her and her facility.

3. The NA should prepare the _____room_____ before the resident arrives.

4. The NA should ask _____questions_____ to find out a resident's personal preferences and _____routines_____.

5. The NA should _____introduce_____ herself to the resident and state her position.

6. The NA should always call a resident by her _____formal_____ name until she tells the NA what she prefers to be called.

7. The NA should try to make sure the new resident feels welcome and wanted. The NA should not _____rush_____ the process or the new resident.

8. The NA can help the resident by explaining daily life in the facility and offering to take the resident on a _____tour_____.

9. New residents must be given a copy of their legal _____rights_____.

10. It is important for the NA to _____observe_____ the new resident in case something important was missed.

11. A resident has a legal right to have his _____personal_____ items that he has brought with him treated carefully.

True or False

12. _F_ A transfer to a new facility or hospital is normally easy for residents to handle.

13. _T_ Residents should be informed of transfers as early as possible.

14. _F_ The resident will usually pack her own belongings for a transfer.

15. _T_ The nursing assistant should introduce the resident to everyone in the new area.

16. _T_ One way that a nursing assistant can involve the resident in the packing process is to show the resident her empty closet.

17. _F_ The NA will write the order when it is time for a resident to be discharged.

18. _T_ OBRA requires that residents have the right to receive advance notice before they are discharged.

2. Explain the importance of monitoring vital signs

Short Answer

1. What might changes in vital signs indicate?

_____condition is worsening_____

2. Which changes should be immediately reported to the nurse?

fever

• respiratory / pulse rate too low

• blood pressure changes

• worse pain / not relieved by pain management

Labeling

For each of the illustrations of thermometers shown below, write the temperature reading to the nearest tenth degree in the blank provided.

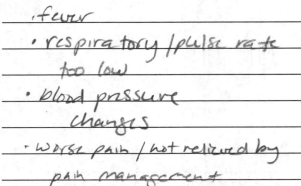

3. _____ 101 °C

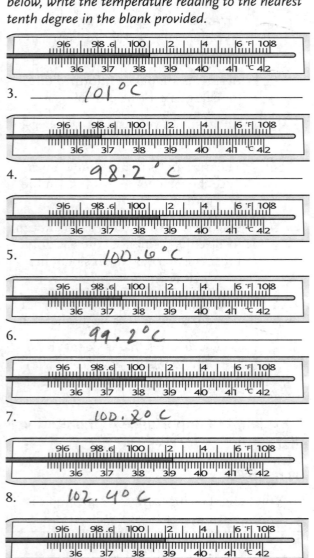

4. _____ 98.2 °C

5. _____ 100.6 °C

6. _____ 99.2 °C

7. _____ 100.8 °C

8. _____ 102.4 °C

9. _____ 102 °C

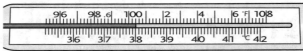

10. _____ 99 °C

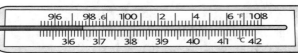

11. _____ 100.2 °C

12. _____ 97.6 °C

Multiple Choice

13. Which of the following is the normal temperature range for the oral method?
    (A) 90.6–94.6 degrees Fahrenheit
    (B) 93.6–97.9 degrees Fahrenheit
    (C) 98.6–100.6 degrees Fahrenheit
    (D) 97.6–99.6 degrees Fahrenheit

14. Which of the following thermometers is used to take a temperature in the ear?
    (A) Temporal artery thermometer
    (B) Rectal thermometer
    (C) Axillary thermometer
    (D) Tympanic thermometer

15. Which of the following temperature sites is another word for the armpit area?
    (A) Rectum
    (B) Temporal artery
    (C) Axilla
    (D) Tympanum

16. Which temperature site is considered to be the most accurate?
    (A) Mouth (oral)
    (B) Rectum (rectal)
    (C) Temporal artery (forehead)
    (D) Ear (tympanic)

17. A rectal thermometer is usually color-coded
    (A) Red
    (B) Green
    (C) Black
    (D) Blue

Basic Nursing Skills

18. Which pulse is most often used for measuring pulse rate?
(A) Apical pulse
(B) Femoral pulse
(C) Pedal pulse
(D) Radial pulse ⟵

19. For adults, the normal pulse rate is
(A) 40 to 60 beats per minute
(B) 60 to 100 beats per minute ⟵
(C) 90 to 120 beats per minute
(D) 20 to 40 beats per minute

20. Inhaling air into the lungs is also called
(A) Inspiration ⟵
(B) Expiration
(C) Rhythm
(D) Pulse

21. Exhaling air out of the lungs is also called
(A) Inspiration
(B) Expiration ⟵
(C) Rhythm
(D) Pulse

22. The normal respiration rate for adults ranges from
(A) 5 to 10 breaths per minute
(B) 12 to 20 breaths per minute ⟵
(C) 25 to 32 breaths per minute
(D) 7 to 11 breaths per minute

23. Why is it important for the NA to observe respirations without letting the resident know what she is doing?
(A) People may breathe more quickly if they know they are being observed. ⟵
(B) People will hold their breath if they know what an NA wants to measure.
(C) The procedure takes less time if the resident is unaware of what is happening.
(D) Observing respirations is a painful process for most people.

24. Which of the following is considered a high blood pressure reading?
(A) 120/79
(B) 130/85 ⟵
(C) 110/70
(D) 100/89

25. Which of the following pieces of equipment is used to measure blood pressure?
(A) Sphygmomanometer ⟵
(B) Reflex hammer
(C) Otoscope
(D) Thermometer

26. The second measurement of blood pressure reflects the phase when the heart relaxes. It is called the _____ phase.
(A) Systolic
(B) Mercurial
(C) Hyperbolic
(D) Diastolic ⟵

27. Blood pressure measurements are recorded as _____.
(A) Rhythms
(B) Fractions ⟵
(C) Decimals
(D) Equations

28. In the _____ phase of blood pressure, the heart is at work, contracting and pushing blood from the left ventricle of the heart.
(A) Systolic ⟵
(B) Mercurial
(C) Hyperbolic
(D) Diastolic

29. A pulse oximeter measures
(A) Blood pressure and heart rate
(B) Blood pressure and pulse rate
(C) Blood oxygen level and pulse rate ⟵
(D) Blood oxygen level and temperature

Short Answer

30. If a resident complains of pain, what questions should the NA ask to get the most accurate information?

• Where is it
• When did it start
• how long lasts / how often
• how severe
• describe it
• what makes it better/worse
• what doing when it started

Name: _____

_____

_____

_____

_____

31. List five things that an NA can do to help reduce a resident's pain.

~~report it~~
- align the body
- back rubs
- warm bath/shower
- bathroom help
- encourage slow/deep breaths
- provide calm /quiet
- be patient

3. Explain how to measure weight and height

Short Answer

1. Why must an NA report any weight a resident loses?

can be sign of illness

2. How many inches are in one foot?

12

Labeling

Looking at each of the readings shown below, determine each resident's weight for numbers 3 to 6 and height for numbers 7 to 10.

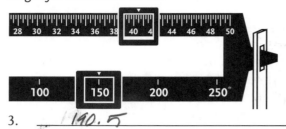

3. _____ 190.5 _____

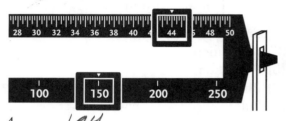

4. _____ 194 _____

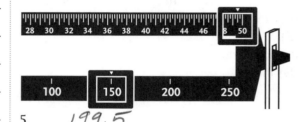

5. _____ 199.5 _____

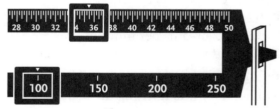

6. _____ 135.5 _____

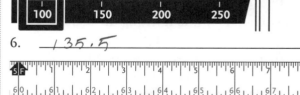

7. _____ 5 ft 2 in _____

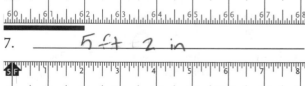

8. _____ 5 ft 8 in _____

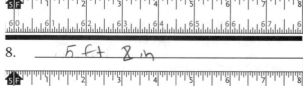

9. _____ 5 ft 5 in _____

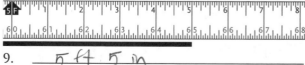

10. _____ 6 ft 3 in _____

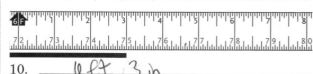

4. Explain restraints and how to promote a restraint-free environment

Multiple Choice

1. The purpose of restraints is to
   (A) Discipline residents
   (B) Make the nursing assistant's job easier
   (C) Restrict voluntary movement or behavior
   (D) Allow ill residents to be left alone for longer periods of time

2. An example of a physical restraint is
   (A) A bed
   (B) A wheelchair
   (C) Medication
   (D) Raised side rails on a bed

3. A chemical restraint is
   (A) Medication used to control behavior
   (B) Medication used to treat illness
   (C) A medical procedure
   (D) A restraint placed on the person's hands

4. What is one reason the use of restraints is now restricted?
   (A) They were found to be too expensive.
   (B) They were abused by caregivers.
   (C) They were difficult for caregivers to use.
   (D) They were not keeping residents occupied for a long enough period of time.

5. A restraint can be used
   (A) For discipline
   (B) When a doctor has ordered its use
   (C) To stop residents from using call lights
   (D) Whenever staff members are busy

6. Restraint-free care means that
   (A) Restraints are used when nurses request they be used
   (B) Restraints are used when necessary for safety
   (C) Restraints are never used for any reason
   (D) Restraints are used with permission from the resident's family

7. Restraint alternatives are
   (A) Measures used in place of a restraint
   (B) Restraints that keep residents in their beds
   (C) Medications used to control a person's behavior
   (D) Periods of confining residents to their rooms

Short Answer

8. When a resident is restrained, he has to be monitored constantly. The resident must be checked often, following facility policy. What care needs to happen at regular, ordered intervals?

   - elimination
   - offer food /fluid
   - take vitals
   - check for skin irritation
   - check for swelling
   - reposition
   - ambulate

5. Define *fluid balance* and explain intake and output (I&O)

True or False

1. __T__ Fluids come in the form of liquids that a person drinks, as well as semi-liquid foods such as soup or gelatin.

2. __T__ The fluid a person consumes is called intake or input.

3. __F__ All of the body's fluid output is in the form of urine.

4. __T__ Fluid balance is taking in and eliminating the same amounts of fluid.

5. __F__ Most people need to consciously monitor their fluid balance.

Matching
Use each letter only once.

6. __E__ Clean-catch specimen
7. __A__ Hat
8. __D__ Routine urine specimen
9. __C__ Specimen
10. __F__ Sputum specimen
11. __B__ Stool specimen

(A) Collection container sometimes put into a toilet bowl to collect and measure samples

(B) Urine and toilet paper should not be included with this specimen

(C) A sample that is used for analysis in order to try to make a diagnosis

(D) Urine sample collected any time the resident voids

(E) Excludes the first and last urine from the sample

(F) This specimen should be collected early in the morning

6. Explain care guidelines for urinary catheters, oxygen therapy, and IV therapy

Matching
Use each letter only once.

1. __E__ Catheter
2. __A__ Condom catheter
3. __D__ Indwelling catheter
4. __B__ Straight catheter
5. __C__ Urinary catheter

(A) Urinary catheter that has an attachment that fits onto the penis

(B) Urinary catheter that is removed immediately after urine is drained

(C) Thin tube used to drain urine from the bladder

(D) Urinary catheter that stays inside the bladder for a period of time

(E) Thin tube inserted into the body that is used to drain or inject fluids

True or False

6. __T__ Oxygen therapy is prescribed by a doctor.

7. __F__ Nursing assistants are usually responsible for adjusting oxygen settings for residents.

8. __F__ A flammable liquid like alcohol is fine to have in a room when oxygen is in use, as long as it is covered.

9. __F__ Smoking is allowed near where oxygen is stored as long as the oxygen is not in use.

10. __T__ Oxygen should be turned off in the event of a fire.

11. __T__ NAs should check the skin around oxygen masks and tubing for irritation.

12. __F__ If a resident has skin irritation around a nasal cannula, the NA should use Vaseline to soften the skin.

Multiple Choice

13. IV therapy allows direct access to
    (A) The joints
    (B) The lungs
    (C) The bloodstream
    (D) The muscles

14. What is the NA's responsibility for IV care?
    (A) Inserting IV lines
    (B) Removing IV lines
    (C) Care of the IV site
    (D) Documenting observations

15. If the fluid in an IV bag is nearly gone, the NA should
    (A) Add saline to the bag
    (B) Notify the nurse
    (C) Replace the bag with a new one
    (D) Reset the pump alarm

7. Discuss a resident's unit and related care

True or False

1. __T__ A resident's room is his home and must be treated with respect.

2. __F__ It is not necessary for an NA to knock and wait for permission to enter a resident's room.

3. __T__ While working in a resident's room, the NA should adjust the temperature to whatever feels comfortable to him.

4. __F__ Urinals and bedpans are normally stored on top of the overbed table.

5. __T__ Call lights must always be answered promptly.

6. __F__ Call lights should be placed wherever it is easiest for the nursing assistant to reach them.

7. __F__ Privacy curtains block sight, as well as sound.

8. __T__ Residents have a legal right to have their privacy protected when receiving care.

9. __F__ Soiled linen should be placed on the overbed table when changing a resident's bed.

10. __F__ It is best for an NA to wait a couple of hours before removing a resident's meal tray.

Multiple Choice

11. If an NA is asked to use a piece of equipment he does not know how to use, he should
    (A) Figure it out as he goes along
    (B) Try to perform the task without using the equipment
    (C) Ask for help
    (D) Refuse to use the equipment

12. Call lights should be placed
    (A) Next to the television
    (B) On the overbed table
    (C) Near the door
    (D) Within the resident's reach

8. Explain the importance of sleep and perform proper bedmaking

Short Answer

1. List five things that can disrupt a resident's sleep.

   • too much sleep during day
   • caffeine intake late in the day
   • wearing PJs all day
   • eating heavy meal late at night
   • refusing sleep meds

2. List three problems that can be caused by lack of sleep.

   • reduced mental function
   • reduced reaction time
   • irritability

Basic Nursing Skills

_____
_____
_____
_____

Multiple Choice

3. Why is it important for NAs to change bed linen often?
   (A) To get residents out of their beds and moving around
   (B) To rotate clean sheets evenly
   (C) To keep NAs' skills up-to-date
   (D) To prevent infection and to promote comfort

4. Why should bed linen be carried away from the NA's body?
   (A) To prevent contamination of clothing
   (B) To keep the linen neat
   (C) To avoid mixing up the linen from different residents
   (D) For proper body alignment

5. When removing dirty linen, the NA should
   (A) Fold it so that the soiled area is outside
   (B) Roll it so that the soiled area is inside
   (C) Gather it in a bunch
   (D) Shake it to remove particles

6. When a resident cannot get out of bed,
   (A) The bed cannot be changed
   (B) The resident will be moved to a stretcher for bed changing
   (C) The nurse will change the bed
   (D) The bed should be raised to a safe height before making it

7. Soiled linen should be bagged
   (A) In the hallway
   (B) In another resident's room
   (C) At the point of origin
   (D) At the nurses' station

8. A bed made with the bedspread and blankets in place is called a(n)
   (A) Open bed
   (B) Stretcher bed
   (C) Closed bed
   (D) Completed bed

9. Discuss dressings and bandages

Fill in the Blank

1. Sterile dressings cover _new, open_ or _draining_ wounds.

2. A _nurse_ changes sterile dressings.

3. Non-sterile dressings are applied to dry, _closed_ wounds that have less chance of _infection_.

Multiple Choice

4. Elastic bandages are also known as
   (A) Non-sterile bandages
   (B) Plastic bandages
   (C) Liquid bandages
   (D) Aseptic bandages

5. One purpose of elastic bandages is to
   (A) Elevate a cast
   (B) Hold a dressing in place
   (C) Cover pressure injuries
   (D) Help with ambulation

6. How soon should an NA check on a resident after applying a bandage?
   (A) 60 minutes
   (B) The next day
   (C) 2 hours
   (D) 10 minutes

8

Nutrition and Hydration

1. Identify the six basic nutrients and explain MyPlate

Short Answer
Write the letter of the correct basic nutrient beside each description below. Use W for water, P for protein, C for carbohydrates, F for fats, V for vitamins, and M for minerals.

1. __P__ Sources include seafood, dried beans, poultry, and soy products.

2. __W__ A person can only live a few days without this.

3. __C__ These help the body store energy.

4. __M__ These add flavor to food and help to absorb certain vitamins.

5. __P__ They are essential for tissue growth and repair.

6. __F__ These may come from olives, nuts, and dairy products.

7. __V__ The body cannot make most of these nutrients; they must be obtained through certain foods.

8. __C__ These provide fiber, which is necessary for bowel elimination.

9. __C__ Examples include bread, cereal, and potatoes.

10. __W__ This is the most essential nutrient for life.

11. __F__ Categories include monounsaturated and saturated.

12. __W__ Through perspiration, this helps to maintain body temperature.

13. __V__ Can be fat-soluble or water-soluble.

14. __M__ These build bones and help in blood formation.

15. __M__ Iron and calcium are examples.

Short Answer
The USDA developed the MyPlate icon and website to help promote healthy eating practices. Looking at the MyPlate icon, fill in the food groups.

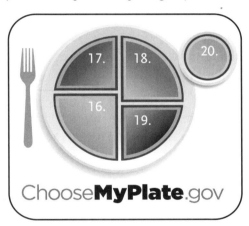

16. __Vegetables__
17. __fruits__
18. __grains__
19. __protein__
20. __dairy__

Multiple Choice

21. MyPlate's guidelines state that half of a person's plate should be made up of
    (A) Grains and protein
    (B) Vegetables and fruits
    (C) Seafood and dairy
    (D) Grains and dairy

22. Out of the following choices, which vegetable color has the best nutritional content?
    (A) Dark green *(circled)*
    (B) Pale yellow
    (C) Dark purple
    (D) Light brown

23. Most of a person's fruit choices should be
    (A) Fruit bars
    (B) Smoothies
    (C) Cut-up fruit *(circled)*
    (D) Fruit juice

24. What kinds of grains are best to consume?
    (A) Refined grains
    (B) White grains
    (C) Whole grains *(circled)*
    (D) Corn grains

25. Which of the following is considered a plant-based protein?
    (A) Salmon
    (B) Eggs
    (C) Sausage
    (D) Beans *(circled)*

26. Oatmeal and pasta are examples of foods made from which food group?
    (A) Vegetables
    (B) Fruits
    (C) Grains *(circled)*
    (D) Protein

27. Most dairy group choices should be
    (A) Full-fat
    (B) 2% fat
    (C) Half & Half
    (D) Low-fat *(circled)*

28. Which of the following foods is considered high in sodium?
    (A) Apple
    (B) Pickle *(circled)*
    (C) Avocado
    (D) Corn

2. Describe factors that influence food preferences

Short Answer

1. Briefly describe some of the foods you ate while growing up. Were there any special dishes that your family made that were related to your culture, religion, or region?

   Growing up I ate a lot of processed food and casseroles. We did eat fruits and vegetables, but they were often canned or frozen. My diet was that of a poor midwesterner.

2. What rights do residents have with regard to food choices?

   They can choose their food and they can refuse food.

3. Explain special diets

Matching
Use each letter only once.

1. __J__   Diabetic diet

2. __G__   Fluid-restricted diet

3. __E__   Liquid diet

4. __A__   Low-fat diet

5. __C__ Low-protein diet

6. __F__ Low-sodium diet

7. __H__ Modified calorie diet

8. __E__ Pureed diet

9. __D__ Soft diet and mechanical soft diet

10. __B__ Vegetarian diet

(A) People who have heart disease or who have had heart attacks may be placed on this diet, which limits the intake of saturated fat.

(B) Health reasons, a dislike of meat, a compassion for animals, or a belief in nonviolence may lead a person to this diet.

(C) People who have kidney disease may be on this diet, which encourages foods like breads and pasta.

(D) This diet consists of soft or chopped foods that are easy to chew. Foods that are hard to chew and swallow, such as raw vegetables, are restricted.

(E) The food used in this diet has been ground into a thick paste of baby-food consistency.

(F) Salt is restricted in this diet.

(G) To prevent further heart or kidney damage, doctors may restrict fluid intake on this diet.

(H) This diet is used for losing weight or preventing weight gain.

(I) This diet consists of foods that are in a liquid state at body temperature and is usually ordered as *clear* or *full*.

(J) Carb counting may be part of this diet, as the amount of carbohydrates eaten must be carefully regulated.

4. Describe how to assist residents in maintaining fluid balance

True or False

1. __T__ Fluid overload occurs when the body is unable to handle the amount of fluid consumed.

2. __F__ If a resident has an NPO order, he can drink water but no other type of fluid.

3. __T__ The sense of thirst lessens as a person ages.

4. __T__ People can become dehydrated by vomiting too much.

5. __T__ A symptom of fluid overload is edema of the extremities.

6. __T__ In order to prevent dehydration, the nursing assistant (NA) should offer fresh fluids to residents often.

7. __T__ One symptom of dehydration is dark urine.

8. __F__ A resident who has swallowing problems should suck on ice chips regularly.

9. __T__ The NA should make sure that the water pitcher and cup are light enough for the resident to lift.

5. List ways to identify and prevent unintended weight loss

Fill in the Blank

1. Encourage residents to __eat__.

2. Give __oral care__ before and after meals.

3. Honor residents' __food__ likes and dislikes.

4. Offer different kinds of foods and __beverages__.

5. Allow enough __time__ for residents to finish eating.

6. Tell the nurse if a resident has trouble using __utensils__.

7. Position residents sitting __upright__ for eating.

8. If a resident has had a loss of __appetite__, ask about it.

9. Record meal/snack __intake__.

Name: _____

6. Identify ways to promote appetites at mealtime

Crossword

Across

1. Should be washed before residents eat

4. Proper position for eating that helps prevent swallowing problems

5. Something that has a positive effect on eating and helps prevent loneliness and boredom

Down

2. Use of eyeglasses, hearing aids, and these should be encouraged

3. Devices that can help residents with eating

6. Noise level should be kept _____ when residents are eating.

h	a	n	d	s					
	e			a					
	n			s					
	t			s					
u	p	r	i	g	h	t			
r				s					
e				t					
s	o	c	i	a	l	i	z	i	n	g
			v		o				
			e		w				

Scenarios

Read each scenario below and make suggestions for making mealtime more enjoyable for the resident.

7. Mr. Leisering comes to dinner in his pajamas. His hair has not been brushed. He is wearing slippers instead of shoes.

    He should be dressed in day clothes, be groomed, and be wearing shoes.

8. Ms. Lopez does not speak very much English. She has not met any of the other Spanish-speaking residents. She comes to meals wrapped in a large sweater and jumps every time she hears trays clattering or when someone raises his voice.

    She should be seated near other Spanish-speaking residents, the temperature should be turned up and the noise should be kept down.

9. Mr. Gaines has dentures, but he says that they cause him pain, so he often does not wear them while eating. It takes him a long time to finish his meals. He has to concentrate so hard on chewing his food that he does not seem interested in talking with anyone around him.

    Mr Gaines should be fitted for new dentures, and perhaps also put on a soft diet.

7. Demonstrate how to assist with eating

True or False

1. *T*   It is important for the NA to identify each resident before serving a meal tray.

2. *F*   The NA should remain standing while feeding a resident.

3. *T*   The resident's mouth should be empty before the NA offers another bite of food.

4. _F_ The NA should refer to pureed carrots as "orange stuff" so the resident knows which food the NA is talking about.

5. _F_ To promote a healthy appetite, the NA should remain silent while helping a resident eat.

6. _F_ If food is too hot, the NA should blow on it for a few minutes until it is cool enough for the resident to eat.

7. _T_ Residents should be sitting upright at a 90-degree angle for eating.

8. _F_ If a resident wants to eat his dessert first, the NA should explain that it is unhealthy and suggest that he begin with his entree.

9. _I_ Alternating cold and hot foods or bland foods and sweets can help increase appetite.

10. _F_ The NA should insist that residents use clothing protectors when eating to help keep clothing clean.

Scenarios

Read each scenario below and describe how each NA can improve his or her technique when assisting at meals.

11. Mrs. Rains, a Catholic resident, asks Carol to join her in a quick prayer before she eats. Carol declines, explaining that she does not believe in God and thinks that prayer is pointless.

The NA should allow
time for prayer b/c
it's not about them.

_____

_____

_____

_____

12. Tracy had a fight with her husband this morning and is in a very bad mood. Mrs. Foster, a friendly resident, tries to make con-

versation as Tracy is handing out meal trays. "I don't have time to talk right now," Tracy snaps at her. "Can't you see how much I have to do?"

Tracy should make
small talk with the
resident then kindly
excuse herself to finish
handing out meal trays.

_____

13. Mr. Parks, a resident with arthritis, can usually feed himself, but today his hands are hurting him so much that he cannot hold the utensils or even his napkin. Carol helps him eat while joking loudly with the other residents that he must be feeling like royalty having someone wait on him hand and foot.

The NA should report
the issue to the nurse,
then help the resident
w/out joking about it.

_____

_____

14. Mr. Correll is recovering from pneumonia. Jamal serves his meal and then watches for a few moments to see if he needs any help. When he determines that Mr. Correll can feed himself, he goes on to help another resident. After he leaves, Mr. Correll starts to feel weak and begins having trouble lifting the utensils to his mouth. He waits for 15 minutes for someone to come back to help him finish his meal.

Jamal should have
stayed to help the
resident as much or
as little as needed

_____

_____

15. While handing out meal trays, Jamal notices that Mr. Gray's diet card indicates a low-sodium diet but his meal tray contains a meal for residents with no restrictions. He assumes the resident's diet must have changed and gives him the tray.

Jamal should have double checked the meal w/ the nurse

_____

_____

_____

8. Identify signs and symptoms of swallowing problems

Short Answer

1. What should the NA do if a resident shows signs of dysphagia?

report to the nurse.

_____

_____

2. Briefly describe three common types of thickening consistencies.

• pudding – semi solid

_____

• honey – honey – consistency, pours slowly

_____

• nectar – thicker than water, like tomato juice

_____

_____

_____

_____

_____

_____

_____

_____

_____

_____

Short Answer

Make a check mark (✓) by all of the correct guidelines for working with residents who require tube feedings.

3. _____ The NA should remove the tube when the feeding is finished.

4. _✓_ During a feeding, the resident should remain in a sitting position with the head of the bed elevated at least 45 degrees.

5. _✓_ Redness or drainage around the opening should be reported.

6. _✓_ The NA is responsible for slowly pouring feedings into the tube.

7. _✓_ The NA should give careful skin care for residents who must remain in bed for long periods to help prevent pressure injuries.

8. _✓_ It is important for the NA to wash his hands before assisting in any way with a tube feeding.

9. _____ After a resident has had a tube feeding, the NA should help the resident lie flat on his back.

9. Describe how to assist residents with special needs

Fill in the Blank

1. Use *assistive* _____ devices such as utensils with built-up handle grips, plate guards, and special drinking cups when necessary.

2. For a resident with a vision impairment, use the face of an imaginary
   _____Clock_____
   to explain the position of what is in front of her.

3. For a resident who has had a stroke, place food in the unaffected, or
   _____Stronger_____,
   side of the mouth.

4. A resident with Parkinson's disease may need help if
   _____tremors_____
   or shaking make it difficult for him to eat.

5. The hand-over-hand approach is an example of a physical
   _____Cue_____
   that can help promote independence.

6. Verbal cues must be short and
   _____Clear_____
   and prompt the resident to do something.

7. If a resident has poor sitting balance, seat him in a regular dining room chair with armrests, rather than in a
   _____wheelchair_____.

8. Put the resident in the proper position in the chair, which means hips are at a
   _____90_____-
   degree angle, knees are flexed, and feet and arms are fully supported.

9. If the resident bites down on utensils, ask him to
   _____Open_____
   his mouth.

10. If the resident pockets food in his cheeks, ask him to chew and
    _____swallow_____
    the food.

Name: _____

9

Rehabilitation and Restorative Care

1. Discuss rehabilitation and restorative care

Multiple Choice

1. What is the goal of rehabilitation?
    (A) To restore the person's intelligence quotient
    (B) To restore the person to the highest possible level of functioning
    (C) To reach the level of functionality of a normal person
    (D) To cure a disease

2. What is the goal of restorative care?
    (A) To diagnose new diseases
    (B) To create new infection prevention policies
    (C) To keep the resident at the level achieved by rehabilitation
    (D) To get the family to visit more often

True or False

3. _F_ The nursing assistant (NA) should ignore any setbacks a resident has so he does not become discouraged.

4. _F_ All residents will enjoy being encouraged in an obvious way.

5. _F_ The NA should do everything for the resident, rather than having him try to do it himself. Doing this will help speed recovery.

6. _F_ The NA should not report any decline in a resident's ability, because all residents in restorative care will have a decline in ability.

7. _T_ Tasks should be broken down into small steps.

8. _T_ It is important for the NA to report any signs of depression or mood changes in a resident.

2. Describe the importance of promoting independence and list ways exercise improves health

Short Answer

1. List nine problems that can result from inactivity and immobility.

    · loss of self esteem
    · depression
    · anxiety
    · boredom
    · pneumonia
    · uti
    · constipation
    · blood clot
    · contractures

2. What does regular ambulation and exercise help improve?

    · skin health
    · circulation
    · strength
    · sleep + relaxation
    · mood
    · self esteem
    · appetite

Rehabilitation and Restorative Care

- elimination
- blood flow
- oxygen level

3. Discuss ambulation and describe assistive devices and equipment

Multiple Choice

1. Assistive devices help residents
   (A) Fight infection
   (B) Make decisions about care
   (C) Perform their activities of daily living
   (D) Communicate

2. Ambulation is another word for
   (A) Walking
   (B) Movement in a wheelchair
   (C) Riding in an ambulance
   (D) Logrolling

3. Supportive devices are used to assist residents with
   (A) Personal care
   (B) Ambulation
   (C) Burns
   (D) Vital signs

4. Safety devices are used for
   (A) Preventing accidents
   (B) Sleeping
   (C) Ambulation
   (D) Incontinence

5. A resident who has some difficulty with balance but can bear weight on both legs should use a
   (A) Walker
   (B) Crutch
   (C) Wheelchair
   (D) Transfer board

6. When helping a resident who is visually impaired to walk, it is important for the NA to
   (A) Keep the resident in front of her
   (B) Let the resident walk beside and slightly behind her
   (C) Walk quickly
   (D) Avoid mentioning stepping up or down

7. Which of the following assistive devices for walking has four rubber-tipped feet?
   (A) C cane
   (B) Quad cane
   (C) Crutch
   (D) Gait belt

8. When using a cane, the resident should place it on his _____ side.
   (A) Left
   (B) Right
   (C) Weaker
   (D) Stronger

Short Answer

9. Choose an adaptive device from Figure 9-6 in the textbook. Describe how it might help a resident who is recovering from or adapting to a physical condition.

   long handled brushes and combs can help residents who have lost mobility and strength to be able to still groom + style their hair.

4. Explain guidelines for maintaining proper body alignment

Fill in the Blank

1. Observe principles of _____alignment_____. Remember that proper alignment is based on a straight _____lines_____.

_____Pillows_____ or rolled or folded ____blankets____ may be needed to support the small of the back and raise the knees or head in the supine position.

2. Keep body parts in natural _____positions_____.
    In a natural hand position, the fingers are slightly ___curled___.
    Use ___bed cradles___ to keep covers from resting on feet in the supine position.

3. Prevent external rotation of _____hips_____. Change _____positions_____ often to prevent muscle stiffness and pressure injuries. This should be done at least every _____2_____ hours.

5. Describe care guidelines for prosthetic devices

True or False

1. __F__ Phantom limb pain is not real pain, so it does not need to be reported to the nurse.

2. __F__ Prostheses are relatively inexpensive and are easy to replace.

3. __T__ A prosthesis is a device that replaces a body part that is missing or deformed because of an accident, injury, illness, or birth defect.

4. __F__ Artificial eyes should be rinsed in rubbing alcohol to prevent infection.

5. __F__ If a prosthesis is broken, it is best for the NA to try to repair it before telling the nurse about it.

6. __T__ When observing the skin on the stump, it is important that the NA check for signs of skin breakdown caused by pressure and abrasion.

6. Describe how to assist with range of motion exercises

Short Answer
For each of the following illustrations, write the correct term for each body movement.

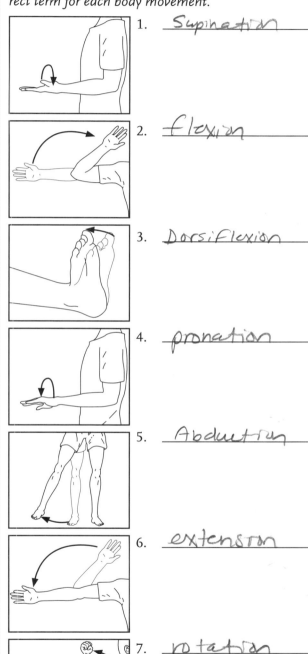

1. Supination
2. flexion
3. Dorsiflexion
4. pronation
5. Abduction
6. extension
7. rotation

Name: _____

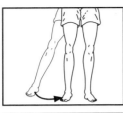

8. ___adduction___

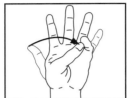

9. ___opposition___

Multiple Choice

10. In what order should the NA perform range of motion exercises?
    (A) He should start from the feet and work upward.
    (B) He should start from the shoulders and work downward.
    (C) He should start at the hands and work inward.
    (D) He should exercise the arms last.

11. If a resident reports pain during range of motion exercises, the NA should
    (A) Continue with the exercises as planned
    (B) Continue, but perform the motion that caused pain more gently
    (C) Stop the exercises and report the pain to the nurse
    (D) Stop the motion for one minute before starting again

12. How many times should each range of motion exercise be repeated?
    (A) At least 6 times
    (B) At least 10 times
    (C) At least 12 times
    (D) At least 3 times

7. List guidelines for assisting with bladder and bowel retraining

Fill in the Blank

1. Residents may need help to restore regular ___routine___ and ___function___.

2. Wear ___gloves___ when handling body wastes.

3. Explain the training ___schedule___ to the resident. Keep a ___record___ of bladder and bowel habits.

4. Encourage plenty of ___fluids___ and foods that are high in ___fiber___.

5. Provide ___privacy___ for elimination, both in the bed and bathroom.

6. Help with ___perineal___ care, which can prevent skin breakdown.

7. Discard clothing ___protectors___ and ___incontinence___ briefs properly.

8. Praise ___successes___ and ___attempts___ to control bladder and bowels.

9. Never show ___frustration___ or ___anger___ toward a resident who is incontinent.

Scenarios

Ms. Potter has been staying at the Cool River Skilled Nursing Center for several months while she recovers from a broken hip. Her recovery is proceeding well, but she has had a problem with urinary incontinence since her injury. Her doctor asks the nurses and nursing assistants on Ms. Potter's unit to assist her with bladder retraining. Below are examples of how three of the NAs help Ms. Potter with retraining. Read each one and state what the NA is doing well and/or what she should do differently.

10. Hannah, a new NA, tries to be very professional about the episodes of incontinence. While she is cleaning the bed, she remains very upbeat and friendly and does not mention the incontinence unless Ms. Potter brings it up.

    ___The NA did well to remain upbeat + professional + not show frustration.___

_____
_____
_____
_____
_____

11. Greta senses Ms. Potter's acute embarrassment and it makes her nervous. Whenever she has to assist Ms. Potter, she speaks very little and does not make eye contact with her. She tries to finish her work as quickly as possible to limit Ms. Potter's discomfort.

Greta could console Ms. Potter, + not be so quick to leave b/c Ms. potter could think She's annoyed w/ her.

_____
_____
_____

12. Takeisha has been very encouraging and positive with Ms. Potter. She has charted her bathroom schedule. She makes sure to be available to help Ms. Potter around the usual times that she needs to go to the bathroom. She responds to her call light quickly.

Takeisha is doing a great job. She is being encouraging, accomodating, and prompt.

_____
_____
_____

10

Caring for Yourself

1. Describe how to find a job

True or False

1. __T__ The internet is a good resource for finding potential employers.

2. __F__ If a potential employer asks a person for proof of his legal status in this country, it means that the employer does not trust the person.

3. __F__ Friends and relatives are the best references to use for a potential job.

4. __T__ A résumé should fit on one page.

5. __T__ A résumé should include a list of educational experience.

6. __F__ A résumé should include a list of a person's religious and political beliefs.

7. __F__ A person's salary information from former jobs may need to be included on a job application.

8. __T__ Identification required by a potential employer may include a social security card.

9. __F__ The abbreviation *N/A* stands for *not answering*. A person uses this abbreviation when he does not want to answer something on a job application.

Short Answer
Make a check mark (✓) next to the descriptions appropriate for job interviews.

10. _____ Wearing jeans

11. __✓__ Looking happy to be there

12. _____ Asking if it is okay to smoke during the interview

13. __✓__ Wearing very little jewelry

14. __✓__ Asking how many hours you would work

15. _____ Bringing your child with you when you cannot find a babysitter

16. _____ Wearing your nicest perfume

17. __✓__ Sitting up straight

18. __✓__ Asking what benefits the employer offers

19. __✓__ Shaking hands with the interviewer

20. _____ Eating a granola bar during the interview so that you are not hungry

21. _____ Asking if you got the job at the end of the interview

2. Describe a standard job description and explain how to manage time and assignments

Short Answer

1. What is a job description?

An agreement between employer + employee, states responsibilities + tasks of job + describes the skills required for the job, who you report to, + salary range.

Name: _____

2. How does a job description protect employ-ers and employees?

protects employees from the facility changing duties w/out notifying them.
protects employers if an employee claims certain duties were not part of their job

3. List five guidelines for managing time.

- plan
- prioritize
- make a schedule
- combine activities
- get help

3. Discuss how to manage and resolve conflict

Multiple Choice

1. When is an appropriate time to discuss an issue that is causing conflict in the workplace?
    (A) When the nursing assistant (NA) decides she cannot take it anymore
    (B) When the NA is upset because some-thing has just occurred
    (C) Right before the NA gives her notice
    (D) When the supervisor has decided on a proper time and place to discuss it

2. When trying to resolve a conflict, the NA should
    (A) Interrupt the other person if the NA might forget what she is going to say
    (B) Sit back in the chair with her arms crossed over her chest
    (C) Take turns speaking
    (D) Yell at the other person if it seems like her point is not understood

3. When discussing conflict, the NA should
    (A) State how she feels when a behavior occurs
    (B) Name-call
    (C) Not look the other person in the eye
    (D) Keep the TV on to fill awkward silences

4. To resolve a conflict, the NA should be pre-pared to
    (A) Compromise
    (B) Quit
    (C) Yell
    (D) Interrupt

4. Describe employee evaluations and discuss appropriate responses to feedback

Short Answer
Read the following and mark whether they are ex-amples of constructive feedback or hostile criticism. Use a C for constructive and an H for hostile.

1. H   "You are a horrible person."

2. H   "If you weren't so slow, things might get done around here."

3. C   "Some of your reports are incomplete; try to be more careful."

4. H   "That was the worst bath I've ever had."

5. C   "I'm not sure that you understood what I meant. Let me rephrase the issue."

6. H   "Where did you learn how to clean?"

7. H   "That was a stupid idea."

8. C   "That procedure could have been performed in a more efficient way."

9. C   "Try to make more of an effort to listen carefully."

10. H   "Stop being so lazy."

5. Discuss certification and explain the state's registry

Multiple Choice

1. The Omnibus Budget Reconciliation Act (OBRA) requires that nursing assistants complete at least _____ hours of initial training before being employed.
    (A) 30
    (B) 50
    (C) 75
    (D) 100

2. OBRA requires that nursing assistants complete _____ hours of annual continuing education.
    (A) 12
    (B) 64
    (C) 75
    (D) 19

3. After completing a training course, nursing assistants are given a(n) _____ in order to be certified to work in a particular state.
    (A) Thesis document
    (B) Residency certificate
    (C) Competency exam
    (D) Apprenticeship

4. Information in each state's registry of nursing assistants includes
    (A) Personal preferences for grooming
    (B) Any findings of abuse or neglect
    (C) Mortgage information
    (D) Special diet requests

6. Describe continuing education

True or False

1. _F_ The federal government requires 20 hours of continuing education each year.

2. _T_ Treatments or regulations can change.

3. _F_ States require less continuing education than the federal government.

4. _T_ In-service continuing education courses help keep an NA's knowledge fresh.

7. Explain ways to manage stress

Multiple Choice

1. Stress is a _____ response.
    (A) Relaxation
    (B) Physical
    (C) Rare
    (D) Supervisory

2. When the heart beats fast in stressful situations, it can be a result of an increase of the hormone
    (A) Testosterone
    (B) Estrogen
    (C) Adrenaline
    (D) Progesterone

3. A healthy lifestyle includes
    (A) Eating when a person is not hungry to calm down
    (B) Exercising regularly
    (C) Smoking a few cigarettes a week
    (D) Complaining about a job

4. Which of the following is a sign that a person is not managing stress?
    (A) Preparing meals ahead of time
    (B) Taking deep breaths and relaxing
    (C) Feeling alert and positive
    (D) Not being able to focus on work

5. Which of the following are appropriate people for an NA to turn to for help in managing stress?
    (A) Residents
    (B) Supervisors
    (C) Residents' family members
    (D) Residents' friends

Short Answer

6. Write out your own personal stress management plan. Be sure to include things like diet, exercise, relaxation, entertainment, etc.

    · diet
    · exercise
    · healthy sleep patterns
    · socialization
    · keeping debt down

Name: _____

_____

_____

_____

_____

_____

_____

_____

_____

_____

_____

_____

_____

_____

_____

_____

7. List five things that you have learned in this course that have surprised or excited you.

- tips on how to interact socially w/ residents

- how to groom others

- PROM exercises

- helping ppl w/ memory loss

_____

_____

_____

_____

_____

8. List two things that you are looking forward to doing when you start working as a nursing assistant.

- Feeding -
I love to care for others, and mealtime can be a great time for a resident to relax and connect

- PROM exercises -
. I find how the body moves and works to be really interesting

_____

_____

_____

_____

_____

_____

_____

Procedure Checklists

2
Foundations of Resident Care

Performing abdominal thrusts for the conscious person		
	Procedure Steps	yes	no
1.	Stands behind person and brings arms under person's arms. Wraps arms around person's waist.		
2.	Makes a fist with one hand. Places flat, thumb side of the fist against person's abdomen, above the navel but below the breastbone.		
3.	Grasps the fist with other hand. Pulls both hands toward self and up, quickly and forcefully.		
4.	Repeats until object is pushed out or person loses consciousness.		
5.	Reports and documents incident.		

_____   _____
Date Reviewed   Instructor Signature

_____   _____
Date Performed   Instructor Signature

Responding to shock		
	Procedure Steps	yes	no
1.	Notifies nurse immediately.		
2.	Puts on gloves and controls bleeding if bleeding occurs.		
3.	Has the person lie down on her back unless bleeding from the mouth or vomiting. Elevates the legs 8 to 12 inches unless signs of injury or fractures exist.		
4.	Checks pulse and respirations if possible.		

5.	Keeps person as calm and comfortable as possible.		
6.	Maintains normal body temperature.		
7.	Does not give person anything to eat or drink.		
8.	Reports and documents incident.		

_____   _____
Date Reviewed   Instructor Signature

_____   _____
Date Performed   Instructor Signature

Responding to a myocardial infarction		
	Procedure Steps	yes	no
1.	Notifies nurse immediately.		
2.	Places person in a comfortable position. Encourages him to rest and reassures him that he will not be left alone.		
3.	Loosens clothing around the neck.		
4.	Does not give person liquids or food.		
5.	Monitors person's breathing and pulse. If breathing stops or person has no pulse, performs CPR if trained to do so.		
6.	Stays with person until help arrives.		
7.	Reports and documents incident.		

_____   _____
Date Reviewed   Instructor Signature

_____   _____
Date Performed   Instructor Signature

84

Name: _____

Controlling bleeding

	Procedure Steps	yes	no
1.	Notifies nurse immediately.		
2.	Puts on gloves.		
3.	Holds thick sterile pad, clean cloth, handkerchief, or towel against the wound.		
4.	Presses down hard directly on the bleeding wound until help arrives. Does not decrease pressure. Puts additional pads over the first pad if blood seeps through. Does not remove the first pad.		
5.	Raises the wound above the level of the heart to slow down the bleeding.		
6.	When bleeding is under control, secures the dressing to keep it in place. Checks for symptoms of shock. Stays with person until help arrives.		
7.	Removes and discards gloves. Washes hands.		
8.	Reports and documents incident.		

_____   _____
Date Reviewed   Instructor Signature

_____   _____
Date Performed   Instructor Signature

Treating burns

	Procedure Steps	yes	no
	Minor burns:		
1.	Notifies nurse immediately. Puts on gloves.		
2.	Uses cool, clean water to decrease the skin temperature and prevent further injury (does not use ice, ice water, ointment, salve, or grease). Dampens a clean cloth and covers burn.		

		yes	no
3.	Covers area with dry, clean dressing or nonadhesive bandage.		
4.	Removes and discards gloves. Washes hands.		
	Serious burns:		
1.	Removes person from the source of burn.		
2.	Notifies nurse immediately. Puts on gloves.		
3.	Checks for breathing, pulse, and severe bleeding. Begins CPR if trained and allowed to do so.		
4.	Does not use ointment, water, salve, or grease. Does not remove clothing from burned areas. Covers burn with sterile gauze or a clean sheet.		
5.	Monitors vital signs and waits for emergency medical help.		
6.	Removes and discards gloves. Washes hands.		
7.	Reports and documents incident.		

_____   _____
Date Reviewed   Instructor Signature

_____   _____
Date Performed   Instructor Signature

Responding to fainting

	Procedure Steps	yes	no
1.	Notifies nurse immediately.		
2.	Has person lie down or sit down before fainting occurs.		
3.	If person is in a sitting position, has him bend forward and place his head between his knees. If person is lying flat on his back, elevates the legs.		
4.	Loosens any tight clothing.		
5.	Has person stay in position for at least five minutes after symptoms disappear.		

6.	Helps person get up slowly. Continues to observe him for symptoms of fainting.		
7.	If person faints, lowers him to floor and positions him on his back. Elevates the legs 8 to 12 inches and checks for breathing.		
8.	Reports and documents incident.		

Date Reviewed _____ Instructor Signature _____

Date Performed _____ Instructor Signature _____

Responding to seizures

	Procedure Steps	yes	no
1.	Notes the time and puts on gloves.		
2.	Lowers person to the floor and loosens clothing. Tries to turn person's head to one side.		
3.	Has someone call nurse immediately or uses call light. Does not leave person except to get medical help.		
4.	Moves furniture away to prevent injury. If a pillow is nearby, places it under his head.		
5.	Does not try to restrain the person.		
6.	Does not force anything between the person's teeth. Does not place hands in person's mouth.		
7.	Does not give liquids or food.		
8.	When the seizure is over, notes time and turns person on left side if head, neck, or spinal injury is not suspected. Checks breathing and pulse. Begins CPR if breathing and pulse are absent and if trained and allowed to do so.		

9.	Removes and discards gloves. Washes hands.		
10.	Reports and documents incident.		

Date Reviewed _____ Instructor Signature _____

Date Performed _____ Instructor Signature _____

Responding to vomiting

	Procedure Steps	yes	no
1.	Notifies nurse immediately.		
2.	Puts on gloves.		
3.	Makes sure head is up or turned to one side. Provides a basin and removes it when vomiting has stopped.		
4.	Removes soiled linens or clothes and replaces with fresh ones.		
5.	Measures and notes amount of vomitus if monitoring resident's I&O.		
6.	Flushes vomit down toilet unless vomit is red, has blood in it, looks like coffee grounds, or has medication/pills in it. Washes and stores basin properly.		
7.	Removes and discards gloves. Washes hands.		
8.	Puts on fresh gloves.		
9.	Provides comfort to resident.		
10.	Puts soiled linens in proper container.		
11.	Removes and discards gloves. Washes hands again.		
12.	Documents time, amount, color, and consistency of vomitus.		

Date Reviewed _____ Instructor Signature _____

Date Performed _____ Instructor Signature _____

Name: _____

Washing hands (hand hygiene)

	Procedure Steps	yes	no
1.	Turns on water at sink, keeping clothes dry.		
2.	Wets hands and wrists thoroughly.		
3.	Applies soap to hands.		
4.	Keeps hands lower than elbows and fingertips down. Lathers all surfaces of wrists, fingers, and hands, using friction for at least 20 seconds.		
5.	Cleans nails by rubbing them in palm of other hand.		
6.	Rinses all surfaces of hands and wrists, being careful not to touch the sink.		
7.	Uses clean, dry paper towel to dry all surfaces of hands, wrists, and fingers. Disposes of towel without touching container.		
8.	Uses clean, dry paper towel to turn off faucet, then disposes of paper towel without contaminating hands.		

_____   _____
Date Reviewed   Instructor Signature

_____   _____
Date Performed   Instructor Signature

Putting on (donning) and removing (doffing) gown

	Procedure Steps	yes	no
1.	Washes hands.		
2.	Opens gown and allows gown to open/unfold without shaking it. Facing back opening of gown, places arms through each sleeve.		
3.	Fastens neck opening.		
4.	Reaches behind and pulls gown until it completely covers clothing. Secures gown at waist.		

5.	Puts on gloves after putting on gown.		
6.	Removes and discards gloves before removing gown. Unfastens gown at waist and neck and removes gown without touching outside of gown. Rolls dirty side in, while holding gown away from body. Discards gown and washes hands.		

_____   _____
Date Reviewed   Instructor Signature

_____   _____
Date Performed   Instructor Signature

Putting on (donning) mask and goggles

	Procedure Steps	yes	no
1.	Washes hands.		
2.	Picks up mask by top strings or elastic strap. Does not touch mask where it touches face.		
3.	Pulls elastic strap over head or ties strings.		
4.	Pinches metal strip at top of mask tightly around nose.		
5.	Puts on goggles.		
6.	Puts on gloves after putting on mask and goggles.		

_____   _____
Date Reviewed   Instructor Signature

_____   _____
Date Performed   Instructor Signature

Putting on (donning) gloves

	Procedure Steps	yes	no
1.	Washes hands.		
2.	If right-handed, slides one glove on left hand (reverse, if left-handed).		
3.	With gloved hand, slides other hand into second glove.		
4.	Interlaces fingers to smooth out folds and create a comfortable fit.		

| 5. | Carefully looks for tears, holes, or spots. Replaces glove if necessary. | | |
| 6. | If wearing a gown, pulls the cuffs of the gloves over the sleeves of gown. | | |

_____ _____
Date Reviewed   Instructor Signature

_____ _____
Date Performed   Instructor Signature

Removing (doffing) gloves

	Procedure Steps	yes	no
1.	Touches only the outside of one glove and grasps other glove at the palm. Pulls glove off.		
2.	With ungloved hand, slips two fingers underneath cuff of the remaining glove at wrist without touching any part of the outside.		
3.	Pulls down, turning this glove inside out and over the first glove.		
4.	Discards gloves without contaminating self.		
5.	Washes hands.		

_____ _____
Date Reviewed   Instructor Signature

_____ _____
Date Performed   Instructor Signature

4
Body Systems and Related Conditions

Caring for an ostomy

	Procedure Steps	yes	no
1.	Identifies self by name. Identifies resident by name.		
2.	Washes hands.		
3.	Explains procedure to resident, speaking clearly, slowly, and directly. Maintains face-to-face contact whenever possible.		

4.	Provides privacy.		
5.	Adjusts the bed to a safe level. Locks bed wheels.		
6.	Puts on gloves.		
7.	Places protective pad under resident. Covers resident with a bath blanket and only exposes the ostomy site. Offers resident a towel.		
8.	Removes ostomy bag carefully and places it in plastic bag. Notes color, odor, consistency, and amount of stool in the bag.		
9.	Wipes area around the stoma with wipes. Discards wipes in plastic bag.		
10.	Washes area around the stoma using a washcloth and warm water. Moves in one direction, away from the stoma. Rinses and pats dry with another towel.		
11.	Places the clean ostomy drainage bag on resident. Holds in place and seals securely. Makes sure the bottom of the bag is clamped.		
12.	Removes bed protector and discards. Places soiled linens in proper container. Discards plastic bag.		
13.	Removes and discards gloves.		
14.	Washes hands.		
15.	Returns bed to lowest position.		
16.	Places call light within resident's reach.		
17.	Documents procedure.		

_____ _____
Date Reviewed   Instructor Signature

_____ _____
Date Performed   Instructor Signature

Name: _____

6
Personal Care Skills

Giving a complete bed bath

	Procedure Steps	yes	no
1.	Identifies self by name. Identifies resident by name.		
2.	Washes hands.		
3.	Explains procedure to resident, speaking clearly, slowly, and directly. Maintains face-to-face contact whenever possible.		
4.	Provides privacy.		
5.	Adjusts the bed to a safe level. Locks bed wheels.		
6.	Places blanket over resident and removes top bedding and top clothing while keeping resident covered. Places clothing in proper container.		
7.	Fills basin and checks temperature (no higher than 105°F). Has resident test water temperature and adjusts if necessary.		
8.	Puts on gloves.		
9.	Asks and helps resident to participate in washing.		
10.	Uncovers only one part of the body at a time. Places a towel or absorbent pad under the body part being washed.		
11.	Washes, rinses, and dries one part of the body at a time. Starts at the head, works down, and completes front first. Uses a clean area of washcloth for each stroke.		

Eyes, Face, Ears, and Neck: Washes face with wet washcloth (no soap) beginning with the farther eye. Using a different area of the washcloth for each eye, washes inner area to outer area. Uses a different area of the washcloth for each stroke. Washes the face from the middle outward, using firm but gentle strokes. Washes ears, behind the ears, and the neck. Rinses and pats dry.		
Arms and Axillae: Washes farther upper arm and underarm. Uses long strokes from the shoulder down to the wrist. Rinses and pats dry. Repeats for other arm.		
Hands: Washes far hand. Cleans under nails. Rinses and pats dry, including between the fingers. Gives nail care. Repeats for other hand. Applies lotion on the elbows and hands.		
Chest: Places towel across chest. Pulls blanket down to waist. Lifts the towel only enough to wash the chest, rinse it, and pat dry. For a female resident: washes, rinses, and dries breasts and under breasts.		
Abdomen: Folds blanket down so that pubic area is still covered. Washes abdomen, rinses, and pats dry. Pulls blanket up to the resident's chin and removes the towel.		

	Procedure Steps		
	Legs and Feet: Exposes far leg and places towel under it. Washes the thigh. Uses long, downward strokes. Rinses and pats dry. Does the same from the knee to the ankle. Washes the foot and between the toes in a basin. Rinses foot and pats dry, making sure area between toes is dry. Provides nail care if it has been assigned. Applies lotion if ordered but not between the toes. Repeats steps for other leg and foot.		
	Back: Helps resident move to the center of the bed, then helps turn him onto his side so back is facing self. Washes back, neck, and buttocks with long, downward strokes. Rinses and pats dry. Applies lotion if ordered.		
12.	Places towel under buttocks and thighs and helps resident turn onto his back. Removes and discards gloves. Washes hands and dons clean gloves.		
13.	**Perineal area and buttocks**: Changes bath water. Places a towel under the perineal area, including the buttocks. Washes, rinses, and dries perineal area, working from front to back, using a clean area of the washcloth for each stroke. After cleaning perineal area, helps turn resident on his or her side, and washes, rinses, and dries buttocks and anal area without contaminating the perineal area.		
14.	Covers resident. Empties, rinses, and dries bath basin. Places basin in dirty supply area or returns to storage. Places soiled clothing and linens in proper containers.		

15.	Removes and discards gloves. Washes hands.		
16.	Puts clean gown on resident and assists with grooming as necessary.		
17.	Returns bed to lowest position.		
18.	Places call light within resident's reach.		
19.	Washes hands.		
20.	Documents procedure.		

_____ _____
Date Reviewed   Instructor Signature

_____ _____
Date Performed   Instructor Signature

Giving a back rub

	Procedure Steps	yes	no
1.	Identifies self by name. Identifies resident by name.		
2.	Washes hands.		
3.	Explains procedure to resident, speaking clearly, slowly, and directly. Maintains face-to-face contact whenever possible.		
4.	Provides privacy.		
5.	Adjusts the bed to a safe level. Lowers head of bed. Locks bed wheels.		
6.	Positions resident in lateral or prone position. Covers resident with blanket and folds back bed covers, exposing resident's back to the top of the buttocks.		
7.	Warms lotion and hands. Pours lotion onto hands and rubs hands together.		

Name: _____

8.	Starting at the upper part of the buttocks, makes long, smooth, upward strokes with both hands. Circles hands up along spine, shoulders, and then back down along the outer edges of the back. At buttocks, makes another circle back up to the shoulders. Repeats for three to five minutes.			
9.	Starting at the base of the spine, makes kneading motions using the first two fingers and thumb of each hand. Circles hands up along spine, circling at shoulders and buttocks.			
10.	Gently massages bony areas. Massages around any red areas, rather than on them.			
11.	Lets resident know when back rub is almost completed. Finishes with long, smooth strokes.			
12.	Dries the back.			
13.	Removes blanket and towel, assists resident with getting dressed, and positions resident comfortably.			
14.	Stores supplies and places soiled clothing and linens in proper containers.			
15.	Returns bed to lowest position.			
16.	Places call light within resident's reach.			
17.	Washes hands.			
18.	Documents procedure.			

_____ _____
Date Reviewed   Instructor Signature

_____ _____
Date Performed   Instructor Signature

Shampooing hair in bed

	Procedure Steps	yes	no
1.	Identifies self by name. Identifies resident by name.		
2.	Washes hands.		
3.	Explains procedure to resident, speaking clearly, slowly, and directly. Maintains face-to-face contact whenever possible.		
4.	Provides privacy.		
5.	Tests water temperature (no higher than 105°F). Has resident test water temperature and adjusts if necessary.		
6.	Positions resident flat in bed. Adjusts the bed to a safe level. Locks bed wheels.		
7.	Places a waterproof pad under the resident's head and shoulders. Covers resident with a bath blanket and wets hair.		
8.	Applies shampoo and massages scalp with fingertips.		
9.	Rinses hair thoroughly. Repeats. Uses conditioner if requested.		
10.	Wraps resident's hair in towel.		
11.	Removes towel and dries face and neck.		
12.	Combs or brushes hair. Dries and styles hair.		
13.	Returns bed to lowest position.		
14.	Places call light within resident's reach.		
15.	Washes and stores equipment. Places soiled linen in proper container.		
16.	Washes hands.		
17.	Documents procedure.		

_____ _____
Date Reviewed   Instructor Signature

_____ _____
Date Performed   Instructor Signature

Giving a shower or a tub bath

	Procedure Steps	yes	no
1.	Washes hands. Places equipment in area. Places bucket under shower chair. Puts on gloves and cleans shower or tub area.		
2.	Removes and discards gloves. Washes hands.		
3.	Goes to resident's room. Identifies self by name. Identifies resident by name. Washes hands.		
4.	Explains procedure to resident, speaking clearly, slowly, and directly. Maintains face-to-face contact whenever possible.		
5.	Provides privacy.		
6.	Helps resident put on nonskid footwear and transports to shower or tub room.		
7.	Puts on clean gloves and helps resident remove clothing and shoes.		
	For a shower:		
8.	Places shower chair in position. Locks wheels. Transfers resident into chair.		
9.	Turns on water. Tests water temperature (no higher than 105°F). Has resident test water temperature and adjusts if necessary.		
10.	Unlocks shower chair and moves it into stall. Locks wheels.		
11.	Stays with resident. Lets resident wash as much as possible.		
12.	Helps resident shampoo and rinse hair. Helps resident wash and rinse entire body, moving from head to toe.		
13.	Turns off water and unlocks shower chair. Rolls resident out of shower.		

	For a tub bath:		
8.	Transfers resident onto chair or tub lift.		
9.	Fills tub halfway with warm water. Tests water temperature (no higher than 105°F). Has resident test water temperature and adjusts if necessary.		
10.	Stays with resident. Lets resident wash as much as possible.		
11.	Helps resident shampoo and rinse hair. Helps resident wash and rinse entire body, moving from head to toe.		
12.	Drains the tub. Covers resident with bath blanket.		
13.	Helps resident out of tub and onto chair.		
	For either procedure:		
14.	Helps resident pat dry. Applies lotion and deodorant as needed.		
15.	Places soiled clothing and linen in proper containers.		
16.	Removes and discards gloves.		
17.	Washes hands.		
18.	Helps resident dress, comb hair, and put on footwear. Returns resident to his room.		
19.	Places call light within resident's reach.		
20.	Documents procedure.		

_____   _____
Date Reviewed   Instructor Signature

_____   _____
Date Performed   Instructor Signature

Providing fingernail care

	Procedure Steps	yes	no
1.	Identifies self by name. Identifies resident by name.		
2.	Washes hands.		

		yes	no
3.	Explains procedure to resident, speaking clearly, slowly, and directly. Maintains face-to-face contact whenever possible.		
4.	Provides privacy.		
5.	Adjusts the bed to a safe level. Locks bed wheels.		
6.	Fills basin halfway with warm water. Tests water temperature (no higher than 105°F). Has resident test water temperature and adjusts if necessary.		
7.	Puts on gloves.		
8.	Soaks all 10 fingertips for at least five minutes.		
9.	Removes hands from water. Washes hands with soapy washcloth. Rinses. Pats resident's hands dry with a towel, including between fingers.		
10.	Places resident's hands on towel and gently cleans under each fingernail with orangewood stick. Wipes stick on towel after cleaning and washes resident's hands again. Dries hands thoroughly, especially between fingers.		
11.	Shapes fingernails in a curve with an emery board or nail file. Finishes with nails free of rough edges. Applies lotion.		
12.	Empties, rinses, and dries basin. Places basin in designated area or returns to storage. Places soiled clothing and linens in proper containers.		
13.	Removes and discards gloves and washes hands.		
14.	Returns bed to lowest position.		
15.	Places call light within resident's reach.		
16.	Washes hands.		
17.	Documents procedure.		

Date Reviewed	Instructor Signature
Date Performed	Instructor Signature

Providing foot care

	Procedure Steps	yes	no
1.	Identifies self by name. Identifies resident by name.		
2.	Washes hands.		
3.	Explains procedure to resident, speaking clearly, slowly, and directly. Maintains face-to-face contact whenever possible.		
4.	Provides privacy.		
5.	Adjusts the bed to a safe level. Locks bed wheels.		
6.	Fills basin halfway with warm water. Tests water temperature (no higher than 105°F). Has resident test water temperature and adjusts if necessary.		
7.	Places basin at comfortable position. Puts on gloves.		
8.	Completely submerges feet in water and soaks feet for 10 to 20 minutes, adding warm water as necessary.		
9.	Puts soap on washcloth. Removes one foot from water. Washes entire foot, including between the toes and around nail beds.		
10.	Rinses and dries entire foot, including between the toes.		
11.	Repeats steps for other foot.		
12.	Applies lotion except for between the toes.		
13.	Empties, rinses, and dries basin. Places basin in designated area or returns to storage. Places soiled clothing and linens in proper containers.		

Name: _____

14.	Removes and discards gloves and washes hands.		
15.	Returns bed to lowest position.		
16.	Places call light within resident's reach.		
17.	Washes hands.		
18.	Documents procedure.		

_____ _____
Date Reviewed   Instructor Signature

_____ _____
Date Performed   Instructor Signature

Combing or brushing hair

	Procedure Steps	yes	no
1.	Identifies self by name. Identifies resident by name.		
2.	Washes hands.		
3.	Explains procedure to resident, speaking clearly, slowly, and directly. Maintains face-to-face contact whenever possible.		
4.	Provides privacy.		
5.	Adjusts the bed to a safe level. Locks bed wheels. Raises head of bed so that resident is sitting up.		
6.	Places towel under head or around shoulders. Removes hairpins, hair ties, and clips.		
7.	If hair is tangled, detangles gently.		
8.	Brushes hair from roots to ends in two-inch sections at a time.		
9.	Styles hair in the way the resident prefers. Offers a mirror to resident.		
10.	Cleans and stores equipment. Puts soiled linen in proper containers. Returns bed to lowest position.		
11.	Places call light within resident's reach.		
12.	Washes hands.		

13.	Documents procedure.		

_____ _____
Date Reviewed   Instructor Signature

_____ _____
Date Performed   Instructor Signature

Shaving a resident

	Procedure Steps	yes	no
1.	Identifies self by name. Identifies resident by name.		
2.	Washes hands.		
3.	Explains procedure to resident, speaking clearly, slowly, and directly. Maintains face-to-face contact whenever possible.		
4.	Provides privacy.		
5.	Adjusts bed to a safe level. Locks bed wheels. Raises head of bed so that resident is sitting up.		
6.	Places towel across resident's chest, under the chin.		
7.	Puts on gloves.		
8.	**If using a safety or disposable razor:**		
	Softens beard and lathers face. Shaves in direction of hair growth, using downward strokes on face and upward strokes on neck. Rinses blade often. Rinses and dries face. Offers mirror.		
	If using an electric razor:		
	Cleans razor. Turns on, pulls skin taut, and shaves with smooth, even movements. With foil shaver, shaves beard with back and forth motion in direction of beard growth. With three-head shaver, shaves beard in circular motion. Shaves chin and under chin. Offers mirror.		
	Final steps:		
9.	Applies aftershave lotion.		

Name: _____

		yes	no
10.	Puts towel and linens in proper container. Cleans and stores equipment.		
11.	Removes and discards gloves. Washes hands.		
12.	Returns bed to lowest position.		
13.	Places call light within resident's reach.		
14.	Documents procedure.		

_____ _____
Date Reviewed Instructor Signature

_____ _____
Date Performed Instructor Signature

Dressing a resident

	Procedure Steps	yes	no
	When putting on items, moves resident's body gently and naturally. Avoids force and overextension of limbs and joints.		
1.	Identifies self by name. Identifies resident by name.		
2.	Washes hands.		
3.	Explains procedure to resident, speaking clearly, slowly, and directly. Maintains face-to-face contact whenever possible.		
4.	Provides privacy.		
5.	Adjusts the bed to a safe level. Locks bed wheels. Raises the head of the bed so the resident is sitting up.		
6.	Dresses resident in outfit of resident's choice.		
7.	Places blanket over resident and removes top bedding and top clothing while keeping resident covered. Takes clothes off stronger side first when undressing. Then removes clothes from weaker side. Places top clothing in proper container.		
8.	Helps resident put on the top. Puts top on weaker arm first, then stronger arm.		

		yes	no
9.	Removes the bath blanket and places it in proper container. Helps resident put on skirt or pants, dressing weaker side first.		
10.	Puts on socks, starting with weaker foot. Puts on shoes, starting with weaker foot.		
11.	Finishes with resident dressed appropriately. Makes sure clothing is right-side-out and zippers and buttons are fastened.		
12.	Returns bed to lowest position.		
13.	Places call light within resident's reach.		
14.	Washes hands.		
15.	Documents procedure.		

_____ _____
Date Reviewed Instructor Signature

_____ _____
Date Performed Instructor Signature

Applying knee-high elastic stockings

	Procedure Steps	yes	no
1.	Identifies self by name. Identifies resident by name.		
2.	Washes hands.		
3.	Explains procedure to resident, speaking clearly, slowly, and directly. Maintains face-to-face contact whenever possible.		
4.	Provides privacy.		
5.	With resident in supine position, removes his socks, shoes, or slippers, and exposes one leg.		
6.	Turns stocking inside-out at least to heel area.		
7.	Gently places the foot of the stocking over toes, foot, and heel. Heel should be in the right place (heel of foot should be in heel of stocking).		
8.	Gently pulls top of stocking over foot, heel, and leg.		

9.	Makes sure that there are no twists and wrinkles in the stocking after it is applied.		
10.	Repeats for the other leg.		
11.	Places call light within resident's reach.		
12.	Washes hands.		
13.	Documents procedure.		

_____   _____
Date Reviewed   Instructor Signature

_____   _____
Date Performed   Instructor Signature

Providing oral care

	Procedure Steps	yes	no
1.	Identifies self by name. Identifies resident by name.		
2.	Washes hands.		
3.	Explains procedure to resident, speaking clearly, slowly, and directly. Maintains face-to-face contact whenever possible.		
4.	Provides privacy.		
5.	Adjusts bed to a safe level. Locks bed wheels. Raises head of bed so that resident is sitting up.		
6.	Puts on gloves.		
7.	Places clothing protector or towel across resident's chest.		
8.	Wets brush and puts on small amount of toothpaste.		
9.	Cleans entire mouth (including tongue and all surfaces of teeth and gumline), using gentle strokes. First brushes inner, outer, and chewing surfaces of upper teeth, then lower teeth. Brushes tongue.		
10.	Holds emesis basin to resident's chin. Has resident rinse mouth with water and spit into emesis basin. Wipes resident's mouth and removes towel.		

11.	Rinses brush and places in proper container. Empties, rinses, and dries basin. Places basin and toothbrush in designated area or returns to storage. Places soiled clothing and linens in proper containers.		
12.	Removes and discards gloves. Washes hands.		
13.	Returns bed to lowest position.		
14.	Places call light within resident's reach.		
15.	Washes hands.		
16.	Documents procedure.		

_____   _____
Date Reviewed   Instructor Signature

_____   _____
Date Performed   Instructor Signature

Providing oral care for the unconscious resident

	Procedure Steps	yes	no
1.	Identifies self by name. Identifies resident by name.		
2.	Washes hands.		
3.	Explains procedure to resident, speaking clearly, slowly, and directly. Maintains face-to-face contact whenever possible.		
4.	Provides privacy.		
5.	Adjusts bed to a safe level. Locks bed wheels.		
6.	Puts on gloves.		
7.	Turns resident on side and places a towel under his cheek and chin. Places an emesis basin next to the cheek and chin.		
8.	Holds mouth open with tongue depressor, or uses gentle pressure on the chin to open the mouth, following facility policy.		

Name: _____

		yes	no
9.	Dips swab in cleaning solution. Squeezes out excess solution. Wipes teeth, gums, tongue, and inside surfaces of mouth, changing swab frequently. Repeats until the mouth is clean.		
10.	Rinses with clean swab dipped in water. Squeezes out excess water first.		
11.	Removes the towel and basin. Pats lips or face dry if needed. Applies lip moisturizer.		
12.	Empties, rinses, and dries basin. Places basin in designated area or returns to storage. Places soiled clothing and linens in proper containers.		
13.	Removes and discards gloves. Washes hands.		
14.	Returns bed to lowest position.		
15.	Places call light within resident's reach.		
16.	Washes hands.		
17.	Documents procedure.		

_____   _____
Date Reviewed   Instructor Signature

_____   _____
Date Performed   Instructor Signature

Flossing teeth

	Procedure Steps	yes	no
1.	Identifies self by name. Identifies resident by name.		
2.	Washes hands.		
3.	Explains procedure to resident, speaking clearly, slowly, and directly. Maintains face-to-face contact whenever possible.		
4.	Provides privacy.		
5.	Adjusts bed to a safe level. Locks bed wheels. Raises head of bed so that resident is sitting up.		
6.	Puts on gloves.		

		yes	no
7.	Wraps floss around index fingers.		
8.	Flosses teeth, starting with back teeth and moving to gum line.		
9.	Uses clean area of floss after every two teeth.		
10.	Offers water periodically and offers a towel when done.		
11.	Discards floss. Empties, rinses, and dries basin. Places basin in designated area or returns to storage. Places soiled clothing and linen in proper containers.		
12.	Removes and discards gloves. Washes hands.		
13.	Returns bed to lowest position.		
14.	Places call light within resident's reach.		
15.	Documents procedure.		

_____   _____
Date Reviewed   Instructor Signature

_____   _____
Date Performed   Instructor Signature

Cleaning and storing dentures

	Procedure Steps	yes	no
1.	Washes hands.		
2.	Puts on gloves.		
3.	Lines sink/basin with towels and partially fills with water.		
4.	Rinses dentures in moderate temperature running water before brushing them.		
5.	Applies toothpaste or denture cleanser to toothbrush.		
6.	Brushes dentures on all surfaces.		
7.	Rinses all surfaces of dentures under moderate temperature running water.		
8.	Rinses denture cup before placing clean dentures in it.		

9.	Places dentures in clean, labeled denture cup with solution or moderate temperature water, or returns dentures to resident.		
10.	Rinses brush. Cleans, dries, and returns the equipment to proper storage. Drains sink and places soiled linen in proper containers.		
11.	Removes and discards gloves. Washes hands.		
12.	Documents procedure.		

_____   _____
Date Reviewed   Instructor Signature

_____   _____
Date Performed   Instructor Signature

Assisting a resident with the use of a bedpan

	Procedure Steps	yes	no
1.	Identifies self by name. Identifies resident by name.		
2.	Washes hands.		
3.	Explains procedure to resident, speaking clearly, slowly, and directly. Maintains face-to-face contact whenever possible.		
4.	Provides privacy.		
5.	Adjusts the bed to a safe level. Locks bed wheels. Lowers head of bed.		
6.	Puts on gloves.		
7.	Covers resident with bath blanket, then pulls down top covers underneath. Asks resident to remove undergarments or assists resident to do so.		
8.	Places a bed protector under resident's buttocks and hips.		
9.	Slides bedpan under hips in correct position (**standard bedpan** positioned with wider end aligned with the buttocks; **fracture pan** positioned with handle toward foot of bed).		

10.	Removes and discards gloves. Washes hands.		
11.	Raises head of bed and props resident into semi-sitting position with pillows. Leaves side rails up (if used) and returns bed to lowest position.		
12.	Makes sure blanket is covering resident. Provides resident with supplies and asks resident to clean hands with wipe when finished.		
13.	Places call light within reach and leaves room until resident calls.		
14.	When called, returns and washes hands. Puts on clean gloves. Raises bed to a safe level. Lowers head of bed. Removes and covers bedpan.		
15.	Provides perineal care if help is needed. Assists with putting undergarments on. Covers resident and removes bath blanket. Discards bed protector and disposable supplies. Places towel and bath blanket in hamper.		
16.	Returns bed to lowest position. Leaves side rails in ordered position.		
17.	Takes bedpan to bathroom and empties bedpan into toilet. Rinses bedpan and empties rinse water into toilet. Flushes toilet. Places bedpan in proper area for cleaning or cleans it according to policy.		
18.	Removes and discards gloves.		
19.	Washes hands.		
20.	Places call light within resident's reach.		
21.	Documents procedure.		

_____   _____
Date Reviewed   Instructor Signature

_____   _____
Date Performed   Instructor Signature

Name: _____

Assisting a male resident with a urinal

	Procedure Steps	yes	no
1.	Identifies self by name. Identifies resident by name.		
2.	Washes hands.		
3.	Explains procedure to resident, speaking clearly, slowly, and directly. Maintains face-to-face contact whenever possible.		
4.	Provides privacy.		
5.	Adjusts the bed to a safe level. Locks bed wheels.		
6.	Puts on gloves.		
7.	Places a bed protector under buttocks and hips.		
8.	Hands urinal to resident or places it if resident is unable. Replaces covers.		
9.	Removes and discards gloves. Washes hands.		
10.	Raises head of bed and returns bed to lowest position. Provides resident with supplies and asks resident to clean hands with wipe when finished.		
11.	Places call light within reach and leaves room until resident calls. When called, returns and washes hands. Puts on clean gloves.		
12.	Discards wipes. Removes urinal. Discards urine and rinses urinal, emptying rinse water in toilet. Flushes toilet. Places urinal in proper area for cleaning or cleans it according to policy.		
13.	Removes and discards bed protector. Removes and discards gloves. Washes hands.		
14.	Leaves bed in lowest position.		
15.	Places call light within resident's reach.		
16.	Documents procedure.		

Date Reviewed	Instructor Signature
Date Performed	Instructor Signature

Assisting a resident to use a portable commode or toilet

	Procedure Steps	yes	no
1.	Identifies self by name. Identifies resident by name.		
2.	Washes hands.		
3.	Explains procedure to resident, speaking clearly, slowly, and directly. Maintains face-to-face contact whenever possible.		
4.	Provides privacy.		
5.	Locks bed wheels and adjusts bed to lowest position. Makes sure resident is wearing nonskid shoes with the laces tied. Helps resident to bathroom or commode.		
6.	Puts on gloves.		
7.	Helps resident remove clothing and sit on toilet seat. Puts toilet paper and disposable wipes within reach. Asks resident to clean hands with wipe.		
8.	Removes and discards gloves. Washes hands. Leaves room or area, leaving call light within reach.		
9.	When called, returns and washes hands. Puts on clean gloves.		
10.	Provides perineal care if help is needed. Assists with putting undergarments on. Places towel in hamper and discards disposable supplies.		
11.	Removes and discards gloves. Washes hands. Helps resident back to bed.		

		yes	no
12.	Puts on clean gloves. Removes waste container and empties into toilet. Rinses container and empties rinse water into toilet. Flushes toilet. Places container in proper area for cleaning or cleans it according to policy.		
13.	Removes gloves and discards them.		
14.	Washes hands.		
15.	Leaves bed in lowest position.		
16.	Places call light within resident's reach.		
17.	Documents procedure.		

_____   _____
Date Reviewed   Instructor Signature

_____   _____
Date Performed   Instructor Signature

Moving a resident up in bed

	Procedure Steps	yes	no
1.	Identifies self by name. Identifies resident by name.		
2.	Washes hands.		
3.	Explains procedure to resident, speaking clearly, slowly, and directly. Maintains face-to-face contact whenever possible.		
4.	Provides privacy.		
5.	Adjusts the bed to safe working level. Locks bed wheels. Lowers head of bed to make it flat. Moves pillow to head of bed.		
6.	Stands on one side of bed with feet shoulder-width apart, facing the head of the bed. Foot closer to the head of the bed points toward the head of the bed. Coworker stands on the other side of the bed.		
7.	Both workers roll up draw sheet to the resident's side and grasp the sheet.		

		yes	no
8.	On count, shifts body weight to front leg and helps resident to move toward the head of the bed.		
9.	Positions resident comfortably, arranges pillow and blankets, and returns bed to lowest position.		
10.	Places call light within resident's reach.		
11.	Washes hands.		
12.	Documents procedure.		

_____   _____
Date Reviewed   Instructor Signature

_____   _____
Date Performed   Instructor Signature

Moving a resident to the side of the bed

	Procedure Steps	yes	no
1.	Identifies self by name. Identifies resident by name.		
2.	Washes hands.		
3.	Explains procedure to resident, speaking clearly, slowly, and directly. Maintains face-to-face contact whenever possible.		
4.	Provides privacy.		
5.	Adjusts the bed to a safe level. Locks bed wheels. Lowers head of bed.		
6.	Stands on same side of bed to where resident will be moved.		
7.	**With a draw sheet:** Rolls draw sheet up and grasps draw sheet with palms up. Puts one hand at resident's shoulders and the other at resident's hips. Applies one knee against side of bed, leans back, and pulls draw sheet and resident on the count of three.		

	Without a draw sheet: Slides hands under head and shoulders and moves toward self. Slides hands under midsection and moves toward self. Slides hands under hips and legs and moves toward self.		
8.	Returns bed to lowest position.		
9.	Places call light within resident's reach.		
10.	Washes hands.		
11.	Documents procedure.		

_____   _____
Date Reviewed   Instructor Signature

_____   _____
Date Performed   Instructor Signature

Positioning a resident on his side

	Procedure Steps	yes	no
1.	Identifies self by name. Identifies resident by name.		
2.	Washes hands.		
3.	Explains procedure to resident, speaking clearly, slowly, and directly. Maintains face-to-face contact whenever possible.		
4.	Provides privacy.		
5.	Adjusts the bed to a safe level. Locks bed wheels. Lowers head of bed.		
6.	Moves resident to side of bed near self.		
7.	Raises far side rail (if used).		
8.	**Turning resident away from self:**		
	Crosses resident's arms over chest. Crosses near leg over far leg. Stands with feet shoulder-width apart and bends knees. Places one hand on resident's shoulder and the other on the near hip. Gently rolls resident onto his side as one unit, toward raised side rail.		

	Turning resident toward self:		
	Crosses resident's far arm over chest and moves arm on side resident is being turned to out of the way. Crosses far leg over near leg. Stands with feet shoulder-width apart and bends knees. Places one hand on resident's far shoulder and the other on the far hip. Gently rolls resident onto his side as one unit, toward self.		
9.	Positions resident properly using pillows or other supports.		
10.	Returns bed to lowest position. Leaves side rails in ordered position.		
11.	Places call light within resident's reach.		
12.	Washes hands.		
13.	Documents procedure.		

_____   _____
Date Reviewed   Instructor Signature

_____   _____
Date Performed   Instructor Signature

Logrolling a resident

	Procedure Steps	yes	no
1.	Identifies self by name. Identifies resident by name.		
2.	Washes hands.		
3.	Explains procedure to resident, speaking clearly, slowly, and directly. Maintains face-to-face contact whenever possible.		
4.	Provides privacy.		
5.	Adjusts the bed to a safe level. Locks bed wheels. Lowers head of bed.		
6.	Both workers stand on same side of bed, one at the resident's head and shoulders, one near the midsection.		

7.	Places resident's arm across his chest and places pillow between the knees.		
8.	Stands with feet shoulder-width apart, bends knees, and grasps draw sheet on far side.		
9.	Rolls resident toward self on count of three, turning resident as a unit.		
10.	Positions resident comfortably with pillows or supports, and checks for alignment.		
11.	Returns bed to lowest position.		
12.	Places call light within resident's reach.		
13.	Washes hands.		
14.	Documents procedure.		

_____   _____
Date Reviewed   Instructor Signature

_____   _____
Date Performed   Instructor Signature

8.	On the count of three, moves resident into sitting position.		
9.	With resident holding onto edge of mattress, puts nonskid shoes on resident.		
10.	Has resident dangle as long as ordered. Does not leave resident alone. Takes vital signs as ordered.		
11.	Removes shoes. Assists resident back into bed by placing one arm around resident's shoulders and the other arm under resident's knees. Slowly swings resident's legs onto the bed.		
12.	Leaves bed in lowest position.		
13.	Places call light within resident's reach.		
14.	Washes hands.		
15.	Documents procedure.		

_____   _____
Date Reviewed   Instructor Signature

_____   _____
Date Performed   Instructor Signature

Assisting resident to sit up on side of bed: dangling

	Procedure Steps	yes	no
1.	Identifies self by name. Identifies resident by name.		
2.	Washes hands.		
3.	Explains procedure to resident, speaking clearly, slowly, and directly. Maintains face-to-face contact whenever possible.		
4.	Provides privacy.		
5.	Adjusts the bed to lowest position. Locks bed wheels.		
6.	Raises head of bed to sitting position. Stands with feet shoulder-width apart and bends knees.		
7.	Places one arm under resident's shoulder blades and the other under his thighs.		

Transferring a resident from bed to wheelchair

	Procedure Steps	yes	no
1.	Identifies self by name. Identifies resident by name.		
2.	Washes hands.		
3.	Explains procedure to resident, speaking clearly, slowly, and directly. Maintains face-to-face contact whenever possible.		
4.	Provides privacy.		
5.	Places chair at head of bed, facing foot of bed, or at foot of bed, facing head of bed. Places chair on resident's stronger side. Removes both footrests close to the bed. Locks wheelchair wheels.		

6.	Raises head of bed and adjusts bed to lowest position. Locks bed wheels.		
7.	Assists resident to sitting position with feet flat on floor. Puts nonskid shoes on resident and fastens.		
8.	Stands in front of resident with feet about shoulder-width apart. Bends knees. Places transfer belt around resident's waist over clothing, and grasps belt on both sides, with hands in upward position.		
9.	Provides instructions to assist with transfer. Braces legs against resident's lower legs. Helps resident stand on count of three.		
10.	Instructs resident to take small steps to the chair while turning back toward chair. Assists resident to pivot to front of chair if necessary.		
11.	Asks resident to put hands on chair armrests and helps resident to lower herself into the chair when chair is touching back of resident's legs.		
12.	Repositions resident with hips touching back of wheelchair. Attaches footrests and places resident's feet on them. Removes transfer belt and checks for proper alignment. Places robe or blanket over lap.		
13.	Places call light within resident's reach.		
14.	Washes hands.		
15.	Documents procedure.		

_____ _____
Date Reviewed   Instructor Signature

_____ _____
Date Performed   Instructor Signature

Transferring a resident using a mechanical lift

	Procedure Steps	yes	no
1.	Identifies self by name. Identifies resident by name.		
2.	Washes hands.		
3.	Explains procedure to resident, speaking clearly, slowly, and directly. Maintains face-to-face contact whenever possible.		
4.	Provides privacy.		
5.	Locks bed wheels. Positions wheelchair next to bed and locks wheels.		
6.	With resident turned to one side of bed, positions sling under resident. Helps resident roll back to middle of bed and spreads out fanfolded edge of sling.		
7.	Positions mechanical lift next to bed, opening the base to its widest point, and pushes base of lift under bed. Positions overhead bar directly over resident.		
8.	Attaches straps to sling properly.		
9.	Raises resident in sling two inches above bed, following manufacturer's instructions. Pauses for resident to gain balance.		
10.	Rolls mechanical lift to position resident over chair or wheelchair. Lifting partner supports and guides resident's body.		
11.	Slowly lowers resident into chair or wheelchair, pushing down gently on resident's knees.		
12.	Undoes straps from overhead bar to sling. Removes sling or leaves sling in place, following facility policy.		
13.	Positions resident comfortably, checking for alignment.		
14.	Places call light within resident's reach.		

15.	Washes hands.		
16.	Documents procedure.		

_____	_____
Date Reviewed	Instructor Signature

_____	_____
Date Performed	Instructor Signature

7
Basic Nursing Skills

Admitting a resident			
	Procedure Steps	yes	no
1.	Identifies self by name. Identifies resident by name.		
2.	Washes hands.		
3.	Explains procedure to resident. Speaks clearly, slowly, and directly. Maintains face-to-face contact whenever possible.		
4.	Provides privacy.		
5.	If part of facility procedure, performs the following:		
	Measures resident's height and weight.		
	Measures resident's baseline vital signs.		
	Obtains a urine specimen if required.		
	Completes the paperwork, including an inventory of all personal items.		
	Helps resident put personal items away.		
	Provides fresh water.		
6.	Orients resident to the room and bathroom. Explains how to work equipment.		
7.	Introduces resident to roommate, other residents, and staff.		
8.	Makes resident comfortable and brings family back in.		
9.	Places call light within resident's reach.		

10.	Washes hands.		
11.	Documents procedure.		

_____	_____
Date Reviewed	Instructor Signature

_____	_____
Date Performed	Instructor Signature

Transferring a resident			
	Procedure Steps	yes	no
1.	Identifies self by name. Identifies resident by name.		
2.	Washes hands.		
3.	Explains procedure to resident. Speaks clearly, slowly, and directly. Maintains face-to-face contact whenever possible.		
4.	Collects the items to be transferred and takes them to the new location.		
5.	Helps resident into the wheelchair or stretcher. Takes her to proper area.		
6.	Introduces new residents and staff.		
7.	Helps resident to put personal items away.		
8.	Makes resident comfortable. Places call light within resident's reach.		
9.	Washes hands.		
10.	Documents procedure.		

_____	_____
Date Reviewed	Instructor Signature

_____	_____
Date Performed	Instructor Signature

Discharging a resident			
	Procedure Steps	yes	no
1.	Identifies self by name. Identifies resident by name.		
2.	Washes hands.		

Name: _____

		yes	no
3.	Explains procedure to resident. Speaks clearly, slowly, and directly. Maintains face-to-face contact whenever possible.		
4.	Provides privacy.		
5.	Measures resident's vital signs.		
6.	Compares the checklist to the items there. If all items are there, asks resident to sign.		
7.	Puts items to be taken onto cart and takes them to pickup area.		
8.	Helps resident dress and then into the wheelchair or stretcher.		
9.	Helps resident say goodbye to the staff and residents.		
10.	Takes resident to the pickup area and assists into vehicle.		
11.	Washes hands.		
12.	Documents procedure.		

_____   _____
Date Reviewed   Instructor Signature

_____   _____
Date Performed   Instructor Signature

Measuring and recording an oral temperature			
	Procedure Steps	yes	no
1.	Identifies self by name. Identifies resident by name.		
2.	Washes hands.		
3.	Explains procedure to resident, speaking clearly, slowly, and directly. Maintains face-to-face contact whenever possible.		
4.	Provides privacy.		
5.	Puts on gloves.		
6.	**Digital thermometer:** Puts on disposable sheath. Turns on thermometer and waits until ready sign appears.		
	Electronic thermometer: Removes probe from base unit and puts on probe cover.		
	Mercury-free thermometer: Holds thermometer by stem. Shakes thermometer down to below the lowest number.		
7.	**Digital thermometer:** Inserts end of digital thermometer into resident's mouth, under tongue and to one side.		
	Electronic thermometer: Inserts end of electronic thermometer into resident's mouth, under tongue and to one side.		
	Mercury-free thermometer: Puts on disposable sheath if available. Inserts bulb end of thermometer into resident's mouth, under tongue and to one side.		
8.	**For all thermometers:** Instructs resident how to hold thermometer in mouth with lips closed.		
	Digital thermometer: Leaves in place until thermometer blinks or beeps.		
	Electronic thermometer: Leaves in place until tone or light signals temperature has been read.		
	Mercury-free thermometer: Leaves in place for at least three minutes.		
9.	**Digital thermometer:** Removes thermometer. Reads temperature on display screen and remembers reading.		
	Electronic thermometer: Reads temperature on display screen and remembers reading. Removes probe.		
	Mercury-free thermometer: Removes thermometer. Wipes with tissue from stem to bulb or removes sheath. Discards tissue or sheath. Reads temperature and remembers reading.		
10.	**Digital thermometer:** Removes and discards sheath with a tissue. Replaces thermometer in case.		

	Electronic thermometer: Presses the eject button to discard the cover. Returns probe to holder.		
	Mercury-free thermometer: Cleans thermometer according to guidelines. Rinses and dries thermometer. Returns to case.		
11.	Removes and discards gloves.		
12.	Washes hands.		
13.	Immediately records temperature, date, time, and method used (oral).		
14.	Places call light within resident's reach.		

_____   _____
Date Reviewed   Instructor Signature

_____   _____
Date Performed   Instructor Signature

Measuring and recording a rectal temperature

	Procedure Steps	yes	no
1.	Identifies self by name. Identifies resident by name.		
2.	Washes hands.		
3.	Explains procedure to resident, speaking clearly, slowly, and directly. Maintains face-to-face contact whenever possible.		
4.	Provides privacy.		
5.	Adjusts bed to a safe level. Locks bed wheels.		
6.	Helps resident to left-lying position.		
7.	Folds back linens to only expose rectal area.		
8.	Puts on gloves.		
9.	Digital thermometer: Puts on disposable sheath. Turns on thermometer and waits until ready sign appears.		
	Electronic thermometer: Removes probe from base unit and puts on probe cover.		
	Mercury-free thermometer: Holds thermometer by stem. Shakes thermometer down to below the lowest number.		
10.	Applies a small amount of lubricant to tip of bulb or probe cover.		
11.	Separates buttocks. Gently inserts thermometer into rectum one-half to one inch. Replaces sheet over buttocks. Holds onto thermometer at all times while taking temperature.		
12.	Digital thermometer: Leaves thermometer in place until thermometer blinks or beeps.		
	Electronic thermometer: Leaves in place until tone or light signals temperature has been read.		
	Mercury-free thermometer: Leaves in place for at least three minutes.		
13.	Removes thermometer and wipes thermometer with tissue from stem to bulb or removes sheath. Discards tissue or sheath.		
14.	Reads temperature and remembers reading.		
15.	Digital thermometer: Cleans thermometer according to policy. Replaces thermometer in case.		
	Electronic thermometer: Presses the eject button to discard the cover. Returns probe to holder.		
	Mercury-free thermometer: Cleans thermometer according to guidelines. Rinses and dries thermometer. Returns to case.		
16.	Removes and discards gloves.		
17.	Washes hands.		
18.	Immediately records temperature, date, time, and method used (rectal).		

		yes	no
19.	Places call light within resident's reach.		

Date Reviewed	Instructor Signature
Date Performed	Instructor Signature

Measuring and recording a tympanic temperature

	Procedure Steps	yes	no
1.	Identifies self by name. Identifies resident by name.		
2.	Washes hands.		
3.	Explains procedure to resident, speaking clearly, slowly, and directly. Maintains face-to-face contact whenever possible.		
4.	Provides privacy.		
5.	Puts on gloves.		
6.	Places disposable sheath over earpiece of thermometer.		
7.	Positions resident's head properly and pulls up and back on the outside edge of the ear. Inserts covered probe and presses the button.		
8.	Holds thermometer in place until it beeps.		
9.	Reads temperature and remembers reading.		
10.	Discards sheath and stores thermometer properly.		
11.	Removes and discards gloves.		
12.	Washes hands.		
13.	Immediately records temperature, date, time, and method used (tympanic).		
14.	Places call light within resident's reach.		

Date Reviewed	Instructor Signature
Date Performed	Instructor Signature

Measuring and recording an axillary temperature

	Procedure Steps	yes	no
1.	Identifies self by name. Identifies resident by name.		
2.	Washes hands.		
3.	Explains procedure to resident, speaking clearly, slowly, and directly. Maintains face-to-face contact whenever possible.		
4.	Provides privacy.		
5.	Puts on gloves.		
6.	Removes resident's arm from sleeve and wipes axillary area.		
7.	**Digital thermometer:** Puts on disposable sheath. Turns on thermometer and waits until ready sign appears.		
	Electronic thermometer: Removes probe from base unit and puts on probe cover.		
	Mercury-free thermometer: Holds thermometer by stem. Shakes thermometer down to below the lowest number.		
8.	Positions thermometer in center of armpit and folds resident's arm over chest.		
9.	**Digital thermometer:** Leaves in place until thermometer blinks or beeps.		
	Electronic thermometer: Leaves in place until tone or light signals temperature has been read.		
	Mercury-free thermometer: Holds thermometer in place for eight to ten minutes.		
10.	**Digital thermometer:** Removes thermometer. Reads temperature on display screen and remembers reading.		
	Electronic thermometer: Reads temperature on display screen and remembers reading. Removes probe.		

	Mercury-free thermometer: Removes thermometer. Wipes with tissue from stem to bulb or removes sheath. Disposes of tissue or sheath. Reads temperature and remembers reading.		
11.	**Digital thermometer:** Removes and discards sheath with tissue. Replaces thermometer in case.		
	Electronic thermometer: Presses the eject button to discard the cover. Returns probe to holder.		
	Mercury-free thermometer: Cleans thermometer with soap and water. Rinses and dries thermometer. Returns to case.		
12.	Removes and discards gloves.		
13.	Washes hands.		
14.	Puts resident's arm back into sleeve.		
15.	Immediately records temperature, date, time, and method used (axillary).		
16.	Places call light within resident's reach.		

_____   _____
Date Reviewed   Instructor Signature

_____   _____
Date Performed   Instructor Signature

Counting and recording radial pulse and counting and recording respirations

	Procedure Steps	yes	no
1.	Identifies self by name. Identifies resident by name.		
2.	Washes hands.		
3.	Explains procedure to resident, speaking clearly, slowly, and directly. Maintains face-to-face contact whenever possible.		
4.	Provides privacy.		
5.	Places fingertips on the thumb side of resident's wrist to locate pulse.		
6.	Counts beats for one full minute.		
7.	Keeping fingertips on resident's wrist, counts respirations for one full minute.		
8.	Washes hands.		
9.	Immediately records pulse rate, date, time, and method used (radial). Records respiratory rate and the pattern or character of breathing.		
10.	Places call light within resident's reach.		

_____   _____
Date Reviewed   Instructor Signature

_____   _____
Date Performed   Instructor Signature

Measuring and recording blood pressure (one-step method)

	Procedure Steps	yes	no
1.	Identifies self by name. Identifies resident by name.		
2.	Washes hands.		
3.	Explains procedure to resident, speaking clearly, slowly, and directly. Maintains face-to-face contact whenever possible.		
4.	Provides privacy.		
5.	Wipes diaphragm and earpieces of stethoscope with alcohol wipes.		
6.	Asks resident to roll up sleeve. Positions resident's arm with palm up. The arm should be level with the heart.		
7.	With the valve open, squeezes the cuff to make sure it is completely deflated.		
8.	Places blood pressure cuff snugly on resident's upper arm, with sensor/arrow on the center of the cuff placed over the brachial artery.		

9.	Locates the brachial pulse with fingertips. Places earpieces of stethoscope in ears. Places diaphragm of stethoscope over brachial artery.		
10.	Closes the valve (clockwise) until it stops. Does not tighten it.		
11.	Inflates cuff to between 160 mmHg to 180 mmHg. If a beat is heard immediately upon cuff deflation, completely deflates cuff. Reinflates cuff to no more than 200 mmHg.		
12.	Opens the valve slightly with thumb and index finger. Deflates cuff slowly.		
13.	Watches gauge and listens for sound of pulse.		
14.	Remembers the reading at which the first pulse sound is heard. This is the systolic pressure.		
15.	Continues listening for a change or muffling of pulse sound. The point of a change or the point that the sound disappears is the diastolic pressure. Remembers this reading.		
16.	Opens the valve to deflate cuff completely. Removes cuff.		
17.	Washes hands.		
18.	Immediately records both systolic and diastolic pressures as a fraction. Notes which arm was used.		
19.	Cleans stethoscope. Stores equipment.		
20.	Places call light within resident's reach.		
21.	Washes hands.		

_____   _____
Date Reviewed   Instructor Signature

_____   _____
Date Performed   Instructor Signature

Measuring and recording weight of an ambulatory resident

	Procedure Steps	yes	no
1.	Identifies self by name. Identifies resident by name.		
2.	Washes hands.		
3.	Explains procedure to resident. Speaks clearly, slowly, and directly. Maintains face-to-face contact whenever possible.		
4.	Provides privacy.		
5.	Makes sure resident is wearing nonskid shoes that are fastened. Starts with scale balanced at zero before weighing resident.		
6.	Helps resident to step onto the center of the scale. Makes sure resident is not holding, touching, or leaning against anything.		
7.	Determines resident's weight.		
8.	Assists resident off of scale before recording weight.		
9.	Washes hands.		
10.	Immediately records weight in pounds (lb) or kilograms (kg).		
11.	Places call light within resident's reach.		

_____   _____
Date Reviewed   Instructor Signature

_____   _____
Date Performed   Instructor Signature

Measuring and recording height of an ambulatory resident

	Procedure Steps	yes	no
1.	Identifies self by name. Identifies resident by name.		
2.	Washes hands.		
3.	Explains procedure to resident. Speaks clearly, slowly, and directly. Maintains face-to-face contact whenever possible.		
4.	Provides privacy.		

		yes	no
5.	Makes sure resident is wearing nonskid shoes that are fastened. Helps resident step onto the scale, facing away from scale.		
6.	Asks resident to stand straight. Helps as needed.		
7.	Pulls up measuring rod from back of scale. Gently lowers measuring rod until it rests flat on resident's head.		
8.	Determines resident's height.		
9.	Helps resident off scale before recording height.		
10.	Washes hands.		
11.	Immediately records height.		
12.	Places call light within resident's reach.		

_____   _____
Date Reviewed   Instructor Signature

_____   _____
Date Performed   Instructor Signature

Measuring and recording urinary output

	Procedure Steps	yes	no
1.	Washes hands.		
2.	Puts on gloves before handling bedpan/urinal.		
3.	Pours the contents of the bedpan or urinal into graduate. Does not spill or splash any of the urine.		
4.	Places graduate on a flat surface. Measures the amount of urine at eye level. Keeps container level and notes amount, rounding up to nearest 25 mL.		
5.	After measuring urine, empties measuring container into toilet. Does not splash urine.		
6.	Rinses graduate and pours rinse water into toilet.		
7.	Rinses bedpan/urinal and pours rinse water into toilet. Flushes toilet.		

		yes	no
8.	Places graduate and bedpan/urinal and container in proper area for cleaning or cleans it according to policy.		
9.	Removes and discards gloves.		
10.	Washes hands before recording output.		
11.	Immediately records the time and amount of urine in output column on sheet.		
12.	Reports any changes in resident.		

_____   _____
Date Reviewed   Instructor Signature

_____   _____
Date Performed   Instructor Signature

Collecting a routine urine specimen

	Procedure Steps	yes	no
1.	Identifies self by name. Identifies resident by name.		
2.	Washes hands.		
3.	Explains procedure to resident, speaking clearly, slowly, and directly. Maintains face-to-face contact whenever possible.		
4.	Provides privacy.		
5.	Puts on gloves.		
6.	Fits hat to toilet or commode, or offers bedpan or urinal.		
7.	Asks resident to void into hat, urinal, or bedpan. Asks resident not to put toilet paper in with the sample. Provides a plastic bag to discard toilet paper separately.		
8.	Makes sure bed is in its lowest position. Provides resident with supplies and asks resident to clean hands with wipe when finished.		
9.	Removes and discards gloves. Washes hands.		

	Procedure Steps	yes	no
10.	Places call light within reach and leaves room until resident calls.		
11.	When called, returns and washes hands. Puts on clean gloves. Provides perineal care if help is needed.		
12.	Takes bedpan, urinal, or hat to the bathroom.		
13.	Pours urine into specimen container, filling it at least half full.		
14.	Covers container with lid. Wipes off the outside with a paper towel. Applies label.		
15.	Places the container in a clean specimen bag.		
16.	Discards extra urine. Rinses hat, urinal, or bedpan and flushes toilet. Places equipment in proper area for cleaning or cleans it according to policy.		
17.	Removes and discards gloves.		
18.	Washes hands.		
19.	Places call light within resident's reach.		
20.	Takes specimen and lab slip to proper area. Documents procedure.		

_____   _____
Date Reviewed   Instructor Signature

_____   _____
Date Performed   Instructor Signature

Collecting a clean-catch (mid-stream) urine specimen

	Procedure Steps	yes	no
1.	Identifies self by name. Identifies resident by name.		
2.	Washes hands.		
3.	Explains procedure to resident, speaking clearly, slowly, and directly. Maintains face-to-face contact whenever possible.		
4.	Provides privacy.		
5.	Puts on gloves.		

	Procedure Steps	yes	no
6.	Opens specimen kit.		
7.	Cleans perineal area, using a clean area of wipe or clean wipe for each stroke.		
8.	Asks resident to urinate into the bedpan, urinal, or toilet, and to stop before urination is complete.		
9.	Places container under the urine stream and instructs resident to start urinating again until container is at least half full. Has resident finish urinating in bedpan, urinal, or toilet.		
10.	Assists as necessary with perineal care. Asks resident to clean his hands with a wipe.		
11.	Covers urine container and wipes off outside with a paper towel. Applies label. Places the container in clean specimen bag.		
12.	Discards extra urine. Rinses urinal or bedpan and flushes toilet. Places equipment in proper area for cleaning or cleans it according to policy.		
13.	Removes and discards gloves.		
14.	Washes hands.		
15.	Places call light within resident's reach.		
16.	Takes specimen and lab slip to proper area. Documents procedure.		

_____   _____
Date Reviewed   Instructor Signature

_____   _____
Date Performed   Instructor Signature

Collecting a stool specimen

	Procedure Steps	yes	no
1.	Identifies self by name. Identifies resident by name.		
2.	Washes hands.		

3.	Explains procedure to resident, speaking clearly, slowly, and directly. Maintains face-to-face contact whenever possible.		
4.	Provides privacy.		
5.	Puts on gloves.		
6.	Fits hat to toilet or commode, or provides resident with bedpan.		
7.	Asks resident not to urinate at the same time as moving bowels and not to put toilet paper in with the sample. Provides plastic bag to discard toilet paper separately.		
8.	Fits hat to toilet or commode, or provides resident with bedpan.		
9.	Makes sure bed is in its lowest position. Provides resident with supplies and asks resident to clean hands with wipe when finished.		
10.	Removes and discards gloves. Washes hands.		
11.	Places call light within reach and leaves room until resident calls.		
12.	When called, returns and washes hands. Puts on clean gloves. Provides perineal care if help is needed.		
13.	Uses two tongue blades to take about two tablespoons of stool and puts it in container without touching the inside. Covers container tightly. Applies label. Places container in clean specimen bag.		
14.	Disposes of tongue blades and toilet paper. Empties and rinses bedpan or container into toilet. Flushes toilet. Places equipment in proper area for cleaning or cleans it according to policy.		
15.	Removes and discards gloves.		
16.	Washes hands.		
17.	Places call light within resident's reach.		

18.	Takes specimen and lab slip to proper area. Documents procedure.		

_____ _____
Date Reviewed   Instructor Signature

_____ _____
Date Performed   Instructor Signature

Providing catheter care

	Procedure Steps	yes	no
1.	Identifies self by name. Identifies resident by name.		
2.	Washes hands.		
3.	Explains procedure to resident, speaking clearly, slowly, and directly. Maintains face-to-face contact whenever possible.		
4.	Provides privacy.		
5.	Adjusts the bed to a safe level. Locks bed wheels. Lowers head of bed and positions resident lying flat on back.		
6.	Removes or folds back top bedding, keeping resident covered with bath blanket.		
7.	Tests water temperature with thermometer or wrist. Water temperature should be no higher than 105°F. Has resident check water temperature. Adjusts if necessary.		
8.	Puts on gloves.		
9.	Places clean bed protector under perineal area, including buttocks.		
10.	Exposes only the area necessary to clean the catheter.		
11.	Places towel under catheter tubing before washing.		
12.	Applies soap to washcloth and cleans area around meatus, using a clean area of the cloth for each stroke.		

13.	Holds catheter near meatus, avoiding tugging the catheter. Cleans at least four inches of catheter. Moves in only one direction, away from meatus. Uses a clean area of the cloth for each stroke.		
14.	Rinses area around meatus. Uses a clean area of the cloth for each stroke. With a clean, dry towel, dries the area around the meatus.		
15.	Rinses at least four inches of catheter nearest the meatus, moving away from the meatus. Uses a clean area of the cloth for each stroke.		
16.	With a clean, dry towel, dries at least four inches of catheter nearest meatus, moving away from the meatus.		
17.	Removes and discards bed protector. Removes towel and places in proper container. Replaces top covers. Removes bath blanket and places in proper container. Places washcloths in proper container. Empties basin into toilet and flushes toilet. Places basin in proper area for cleaning or cleans and stores according to policy.		
18.	Removes and discards gloves.		
19.	Washes hands.		
20.	Returns bed to lowest position.		
21.	Places call light within resident's reach.		
22.	Documents procedure.		

_____   _____
Date Reviewed   Instructor Signature

_____   _____
Date Performed   Instructor Signature

Emptying the catheter drainage bag

	Procedure Steps	yes	no
1.	Identifies self by name. Identifies resident by name.		
2.	Washes hands.		
3.	Explains procedure to resident, speaking clearly, slowly, and directly. Maintains face-to-face contact whenever possible.		
4.	Provides privacy.		
5.	Puts on gloves.		
6.	Places measuring container on paper towel on floor.		
7.	Opens drain or spout on bag so urine flows into graduate. Does not let spout or clamp touch graduate.		
8.	Closes spout and cleans it. Replaces drain in its holder on the bag.		
9.	Places graduate on flat surface in bathroom. Notes amount and appearance of urine and empties it into toilet. Flushes toilet.		
10.	Cleans and stores graduate properly. Discards paper towels.		
11.	Removes and discards gloves.		
12.	Washes hands.		
13.	Documents procedure.		

_____   _____
Date Reviewed   Instructor Signature

_____   _____
Date Performed   Instructor Signature

Making an occupied bed

	Procedure Steps	yes	no
1.	Identifies self by name. Identifies resident by name.		
2.	Washes hands.		
3.	Explains procedure to resident, speaking clearly, slowly, and directly. Maintains face-to-face contact whenever possible.		

4.	Provides privacy.		
5.	Places clean linen on clean surface within reach (e.g., bedside stand, overbed table, or chair).		
6.	Adjusts the bed to a safe working level, usually waist high. Lowers head of bed. Locks bed wheels.		
7.	Puts on gloves.		
8.	Loosens top linen from working side. Unfolds bath blanket over top sheet to cover resident and removes top sheet.		
9.	Raises side rail on far side of bed and turns resident onto her side, away from self, toward raised side rail.		
10.	Loosens bottom soiled linen, mattress pad, and protector on working side.		
11.	Rolls bottom soiled linen toward resident, soiled side inside. Tucks it snugly against the resident's back.		
12.	Places and tucks in clean bottom linen, finishing with no wrinkles. Makes hospital corners if necessary.		
13.	Smoothes bottom sheet out toward the resident. Rolls extra material toward resident and tucks it under resident's body.		
14.	Places waterproof bed protector, if using, and centers it. Tucks side near self under mattress and smoothes it out toward resident.		
15.	Places draw sheet if using. Smoothes and tucks as with other bedding.		
16.	Raises side rail nearest self and lowers side rail on other side of bed. Assists resident to turn onto clean bottom sheet.		

17.	Loosens soiled linen. Rolls linen from head to foot of bed, avoiding contact with skin or clothes. Places it in hamper or bag.		
18.	Pulls through and tucks in clean bottom linen just like other side, finishing with bottom sheet free of wrinkles.		
19.	Asks resident to turn onto her back, keeping resident covered. Raises side rail.		
20.	Unfolds top sheet and places it over resident. Asks resident to hold onto top sheet and slips blanket or old sheet out from underneath. Puts it in hamper or bag.		
21.	Places a blanket over the top sheet, matching the top edges. Tucks bottom edges of top sheet and blanket under mattress, making hospital corners on each side. Loosens top linens over resident's feet. Folds top sheet over the blanket about six inches.		
22.	Removes pillows and pillowcases. Places pillowcases in hamper or bag.		
23.	Removes and discards gloves. Washes hands.		
24.	Places clean pillowcases on pillows. Places them under resident's head with open end away from door.		
25.	Returns bed to lowest position. Leaves side rails in ordered position.		
26.	Places call light within resident's reach.		
27.	Takes hamper or bag to proper area.		
28.	Washes hands.		
29.	Documents procedure.		

Date Reviewed	Instructor Signature
Date Performed	Instructor Signature

Date Reviewed	Instructor Signature
Date Performed	Instructor Signature

Making an unoccupied bed

	Procedure Steps	yes	no
1.	Washes hands.		
2.	Places clean linen on clean surface within reach (e.g., bedside stand, overbed table, or chair).		
3.	Adjusts the bed to a safe level. Puts bed in flattest position. Locks bed wheels.		
4.	Puts on gloves.		
5.	Loosens soiled linen and rolls it from head to foot of bed. Avoids contact with skin or clothes. Places it in a hamper or bag.		
6.	Removes and discards gloves. Washes hands.		
7.	Remakes bed, spreading mattress pad and bottom sheet, tucking under mattress. Makes hospital corners. Puts on mattress protector and draw sheet, smoothes, and tucks under sides of bed.		
8.	Places top sheet and blanket, centering them. Tucks under end of bed and makes hospital corners. Folds down top sheet over the blanket about six inches.		
9.	Removes pillows and pillowcases. Puts on clean pillowcases. Replaces pillows.		
10.	Returns bed to its lowest position.		
11.	Takes hamper or bag to proper area.		
12.	Washes hands.		
13.	Documents procedure.		

Changing a dry dressing using non-sterile technique

	Procedure Steps	yes	no
1.	Identifies self by name. Identifies resident by name.		
2.	Washes hands.		
3.	Explains procedure to resident, speaking clearly, slowly, and directly. Maintains face-to-face contact whenever possible.		
4.	Provides privacy.		
5.	Cuts pieces of tape long enough to secure the dressing. Opens gauze package without touching the gauze. Places open package on flat surface.		
6.	Puts on gloves.		
7.	Removes soiled dressing gently by peeling tape toward wound. Lifts dressing off the wound and observes dressing for odor or drainage. Notes color and size of the wound. Discards used dressing in proper container. Removes and discards gloves in plastic bag. Washes hands.		
8.	Puts on new gloves.		
9.	Applies clean gauze to wound. Tapes gauze in place. Discards supplies.		
10.	Removes and discards gloves.		
11.	Washes hands.		
12.	Places call light within resident's reach.		
13.	Documents procedure.		

Date Reviewed	Instructor Signature
Date Performed	Instructor Signature

8
Nutrition and Hydration

Serving fresh water

	Procedure Steps	yes	no
1.	Identifies self by name. Identifies resident by name.		
2.	Washes hands.		
3.	Puts on gloves.		
4.	Scoops ice into water pitcher. Adds fresh water.		
5.	Uses and stores ice scoop properly.		
6.	Takes pitcher to resident. Pours glass of water for resident and leaves pitcher and glass at bedside.		
7.	Makes sure pitcher and glass are light enough for resident to lift. Leaves a straw if resident wants one.		
8.	Places call light within resident's reach.		
9.	Removes and discards gloves.		
10.	Washes hands.		

_____   _____
Date Reviewed   Instructor Signature

_____   _____
Date Performed   Instructor Signature

Feeding a resident

	Procedure Steps	yes	no
1.	Identifies self by name. Identifies resident by name.		
2.	Washes hands.		
3.	Explains procedure to resident, speaking clearly, slowly, and directly. Maintains face-to-face contact whenever possible.		
4.	Provides privacy.		
5.	Picks up diet card and asks resident to state his name, or checks ID a different way. Verifies that resident has received the right tray.		
6.	Raises the head of the bed. Makes sure resident is in an upright sitting position.		
7.	Adjusts bed height to seat self at resident's eye level. Locks bed wheels.		
8.	Places meal tray where it can be easily seen by resident, such as on overbed table.		
9.	Helps resident clean hands if needed.		
10.	Helps resident to put on clothing protector if desired.		
11.	Sits facing resident, at resident's eye level, on the stronger side.		
12.	Tells resident what foods are on the plate and offers a drink of beverage. Asks what resident would like to eat first.		
13.	Offers the food in bite-sized pieces, telling resident content of each bite offered. Alternates types of food offered, allowing for resident's preferences. Makes sure resident's mouth is empty before next bite of food or sip of beverage.		
14.	Offers drinks of beverage throughout the meal.		
15.	Talks with resident during meal.		
16.	Wipes food from resident's mouth and hands as necessary during the meal. Wipes again at the end of the meal.		
17.	Removes clothing protector if used. Places it and used washcloths or wipes in the proper containers.		
18.	Removes food tray, checking for personal items. Places tray in proper area.		

19.	Returns bed to lowest position.		
20.	Places call light within resident's reach.		
21.	Washes hands.		
22.	Documents procedure.		

_____   _____
Date Reviewed   Instructor Signature

_____   _____
Date Performed   Instructor Signature

9
Rehabilitation and Restorative Care

Assisting a resident to ambulate		
	Procedure Steps	yes	no
1.	Identifies self by name. Identifies resident by name.		
2.	Washes hands.		
3.	Explains procedure to resident, speaking clearly, slowly, and directly. Maintains face-to-face contact whenever possible.		
4.	Provides privacy.		
5.	Adjusts the bed to lowest position. Locks bed wheels. Assists resident into sitting position with feet flat on the floor. Adjusts bed height if needed. Puts nonskid footwear on resident and fastens.		
6.	Stands in front of and faces resident with feet shoulder-width apart.		
7.	Places gait belt around resident's waist over clothing. Grasps belt on both sides, with hands in upward position. Braces resident's lower extremities and bends knees.		

8.	Has resident lean forward, push down on bed with his hands, and stand on count of three. While counting, begins to rock. On three, grasping gait belt and moving upward, rocks weight onto back foot. Slowly helps resident to stand.		
9.	Walks slightly behind and to one side of resident for the entire distance while holding on to gait belt. Asks resident to look forward, not down at the floor.		
10.	Removes gait belt and returns resident to bed or a chair. Positions resident comfortably and checks alignment. Leaves bed in lowest position.		
11.	Places call light within resident's reach.		
12.	Washes hands.		
13.	Documents procedure.		

_____   _____
Date Reviewed   Instructor Signature

_____   _____
Date Performed   Instructor Signature

Assisting with ambulation for a resident using a cane, walker, or crutches		
	Procedure Steps	yes	no
1.	Identifies self by name. Identifies resident by name.		
2.	Washes hands.		
3.	Explains procedure to resident, speaking clearly, slowly, and directly. Maintains face-to-face contact whenever possible.		
4.	Provides privacy.		
5.	Adjusts the bed to lowest position so that feet are flat on the floor. Locks bed wheels. Puts nonskid footwear on resident and fastens.		

6.	Stands in front of and faces resident with feet shoulder-width apart.		
7.	Places gait belt around resident's waist over clothing. Grasps belt on both sides, with hands in upward position. Braces resident's lower extremities and bends knees. Assists resident to stand.		
8.	Helps as needed with ambulation with cane, walker, or crutches, walking slightly behind or on the weak side of resident. Holds gait belt.		
9.	Watches for obstacles in the resident's path.		
10.	Lets the resident set the pace, encouraging rest as necessary.		
11.	Removes gait belt and returns resident to bed or a chair. Positions resident comfortably and checks alignment. Leaves bed in lowest position.		
12.	Places call light within resident's reach.		
13.	Washes hands.		
14.	Documents procedure.		

_____   _____
Date Reviewed   Instructor Signature

_____   _____
Date Performed   Instructor Signature

Assisting with passive range of motion exercises

	Procedure Steps	yes	no
1.	Identifies self by name. Identifies resident by name.		
2.	Washes hands.		
3.	Explains procedure to resident, speaking clearly, slowly, and directly. Maintains face-to-face contact whenever possible.		
4.	Provides privacy.		
5.	Adjusts the bed to a safe level. Locks bed wheels.		
6.	Positions resident in supine position.		
7.	Repeats each exercise at least three times.		
8.	**Shoulder:** Performs the following movements properly, supporting the resident's arm at the elbow and wrist by placing one hand under the elbow and the other hand under the wrist:		
	1. Extension		
	2. Flexion		
	3. Abduction		
	4. Adduction		
	Elbow: Performs the following movements properly, holding the wrist with one hand and holding the elbow with the other:		
	1. Flexion		
	2. Extension		
	3. Pronation		
	4. Supination		
	Wrist: Performs the following movements properly, holding the wrist with one hand and using the fingers of the other hand to help the joint through the motions:		
	1. Flexion		
	2. Dorsiflexion		
	3. Radial flexion		
	4. Ulnar flexion		
	Thumb: Performs the following movements properly:		
	1. Abduction		
	2. Adduction		

Name: _____

3. Opposition			
4. Flexion			
5. Extension			
Fingers:			
Performs the following movements properly:			
1. Flexion			
2. Extension			
3. Abduction			
4. Adduction			
Hip:			
Performs the following movements properly, placing one hand under the knee and one under the ankle:			
1. Abduction			
2. Adduction			
3. Internal rotation			
4. External rotation			
Knees:			
Performs the following movements properly, placing one hand under the knee and one under the ankle:			
1. Flexion			
2. Extension			
Ankles:			
Performs the following movements properly, supporting the foot and ankle:			
1. Dorsiflexion			
2. Plantar flexion			
3. Supination			
4. Pronation			
Toes:			
Performs the following movements properly:			
1. Flexion			
2. Extension			
3. Abduction			

	When all exercises are completed:		
9.	Returns resident to comfortable position and covers as appropriate. Returns bed to lowest position.		
10.	Places call light within resident's reach.		
11.	Washes hands.		
12.	Documents procedure. Notes any decrease in range of motion or any pain experienced by the resident. Notifies nurse if increased stiffness or physical resistance is noted.		

_____   _____
Date Reviewed   Instructor Signature

_____   _____
Date Performed   Instructor Signature

Practice Exam

Taking an Exam

After a nursing assistant has completed an approved training program in her state, she is given a competency evaluation (a certification exam or test) in order to be certified to work in that state. This exam usually consists of both a written evaluation and a skills evaluation. Here are some guidelines for taking exams to help you feel better prepared.

Your physical condition affects your mental abilities. Before taking an exam, get plenty of sleep and watch what you eat and drink. On the day of the exam, eat a healthy breakfast. It can be hard to think if you are hungry or if you did not eat a balanced breakfast. Avoid foods that contain simple sugars like soda and doughnuts.

Being in good physical shape allows for more blood to get to the brain. If you get regular physical exercise, your body and mind uses oxygen more effectively. Even exercising a few days before an exam can make a noticeable difference in thinking abilities.

When taking the exam, listen carefully to any instructions given. Be sure to read the directions. When taking a multiple-choice test, first eliminate answers you know are wrong. Since your first choice is usually correct, do not change your answers unless you are sure of the correction.

Do not spend too much time on any one question. If you do not understand it, move on and go back if time allows. Remember to leave that question blank on your answer sheet. Be careful to answer the next question in the proper space. When you are finished with the test, review your answers. For the skills portion of the exam, review the procedures in the book and any notes you may have taken from lectures.

Many testing companies have information available on their websites regarding how to reschedule exams, supplies needed for a particular skill, what to bring to the testing site, and what to wear on the day of the exam. You will need to know which company performs the testing for your state.

Some of the testing sites are listed below. Their websites have more information about the testing process.

- Pearson VUE (pearsonvue.com)

- D&S Diversified Technologies/Headmaster (hdmaster.com)

- Prometric (prometric.com)

Remember that being nervous is natural. Most people get nervous before and during a test. A little stress can actually help you focus and make you more alert. A few deep breaths can help calm you down. Try it. Most importantly, believe in yourself. You can do it!

Practice Exam

1. When a resident refuses to let the nursing assistant take her blood pressure, the nursing assistant should
   (A) Let the resident know that she must have it taken to prevent a serious illness
   (B) Take the resident's blood pressure anyway and agree to report the refusal later
   (C) Promise the resident a gift if she allows her blood pressure to be measured
   (D) Report this to the nurse

2. One task commonly assigned to nursing assistants is
   (A) Inserting and removing tubes
   (B) Changing sterile dressings
   (C) Helping residents with elimination needs
   (D) Prescribing medications to residents

3. A nursing assistant may share a resident's medical information with which of the following?
   (A) The resident's family
   (B) Other members of the healthcare team
   (C) The nursing assistant's family
   (D) The resident's roommate

120

4. To best communicate with a resident who has a hearing impairment, the nursing assistant should
   (A) Use short sentences and simple words
   (B) Shout the words slowly
   (C) Approach the resident from behind
   (D) Raise the pitch of her voice

5. If a nursing assistant suspects that a resident is being abused, she should
   (A) Ask the resident if he thinks he is being abused
   (B) Call the resident's family immediately to report the possible abuse
   (C) Report it to the nurse immediately
   (D) Check with the resident's roommate to see if he has noticed anything

6. An ombudsman is a person who
   (A) Is in charge of hiring facility staff
   (B) Teaches nursing assistants how to perform range of motion exercises
   (C) Is a legal advocate for residents and helps protect their rights
   (D) Creates special diets for residents who are ill

7. To best respond to a resident with Alzheimer's disease who is repeating a question over and over again, the nursing assistant should
   (A) Answer questions each time they are asked, using the same words
   (B) Try to silence the resident
   (C) Ask the resident to stop repeating herself
   (D) Explain to the resident that she just asked that question

8. With regard to a resident's toenails, a nursing assistant should
   (A) Never cut them
   (B) Cut them when the resident requests it
   (C) Cut them weekly
   (D) File them into rounded edges — possibly right

9. When providing personal care, the nursing assistant should
   (A) Make sure the resident remains silent
   (B) Provide privacy for the resident
   (C) Tell the resident about other residents' conditions to distract him
   (D) Discuss her personal problems

10. Generally speaking, the last sense to leave a dying person is the sense of
   (A) Sight
   (B) Taste
   (C) Smell
   (D) Hearing

11. Which temperature site is considered the most accurate?
   (A) Rectum (rectal)
   (B) Mouth (oral)
   (C) Armpit (axillary)
   (D) Ear (tympanic)

12. How should a standard bedpan be positioned?
   (A) It should be positioned however the resident prefers.
   (B) The wider end should be aligned with the resident's buttocks.
   (C) The smaller end should be aligned with the resident's buttocks.
   (D) The smaller end should be facing the resident's head.

13. A resident tells a nursing assistant that she is scared of dying. Which would be the best response by the nursing assistant (NA)?
   (A) The NA can offer to call her minister to see if he can visit the resident.
   (B) The NA can listen quietly and ask questions when appropriate.
   (C) The NA can reassure the resident that she is not dying soon.
   (D) The NA can suggest other medications that might help with the resident's condition.

14. To prevent dehydration, a nursing assistant should
   (A) Discourage fluids before bedtime
   (B) Withhold fluids so the resident will be really thirsty
   (C) Offer fresh water and other fluids often
   (D) Wake the resident during the night to offer fluids

15. When giving perineal care to a female resident, a nursing assistant should
    (A) Wipe from front to back
    (B) Wipe from back to front
    (C) Use the same section of the washcloth for cleaning each part
    (D) Wash the anal area before the perineal area

16. If a nursing assistant sees a resident masturbating, the nursing assistant should
    (A) Ask the charge nurse what she is legally allowed to do
    (B) Provide privacy for the resident
    (C) Suggest that nighttime might be better for masturbating
    (D) Ask the resident to stop masturbating

17. In what order should range of motion exercises be performed?
    (A) Start from the feet and work up.
    (B) Start from the shoulders and work down.
    (C) Exercise the arms and legs first.
    (D) Exercise the arms and legs last.

18. A nursing assistant must wear gloves when
    (A) Combing a resident's hair
    (B) Feeding a resident
    (C) Performing oral care
    (D) Performing range of motion exercises

19. To best communicate with a resident who has a vision impairment, the nursing assistant should
    (A) Rearrange furniture without telling the resident
    (B) Identify herself when she enters the room
    (C) Keep the lighting low at all times
    (D) Touch the resident before identifying herself

20. The first stage of a pressure injury may have skin that is this color:
    (A) Yellow
    (B) Freckled
    (C) Red
    (D) Blue

21. Which one of the following statements is generally true of the normal aging process and late adulthood (65 years and older)?
    (A) People become helpless and lonely.
    (B) People become incontinent.
    (C) People develop Alzheimer's disease.
    (D) People remain active and engaged.

22. Abdominal thrusts help
    (A) Stop bleeding
    (B) Remove a blockage from an airway
    (C) Reduce the risk of falls
    (D) Stop a heart attack

23. Which of the following is a way to prevent unintended weight loss?
    (A) Insisting that residents eat whatever food is offered to them
    (B) Asking residents to swallow more quickly
    (C) Offering gifts to residents who finish their meals
    (D) Honoring food likes and dislikes

24. Which of the following is a way for a nursing assistant to use proper body mechanics while working?
    (A) Bending his knees while lifting
    (B) Standing with his feet close together while lifting
    (C) Holding objects far away from his body when carrying them
    (D) Twisting at the waist when he is moving an object

25. What would be the best way for a nursing assistant to promote a resident's independence and dignity during bowel or bladder retraining?
    (A) Rushing the resident during elimination
    (B) Providing privacy for elimination
    (C) Criticizing a resident when he has a setback to help keep him motivated
    (D) Withholding fluids when the resident is incontinent

26. A resident tells a nursing assistant that he wants to wear his gray sweater. The nursing assistant should
  (A) Tell him that she has already picked out his clothes for the day
  (B) Assist him in getting dressed in his gray sweater
  (C) Tell him that his gray sweater does not match his pants and ask him to pick something else
  (D) Tell him that she likes his blue sweater better

27. When donning (putting on) personal protective equipment (PPE), which of the following should be donned first?
  (A) Mask
  (B) Gown
  (C) Gloves
  (D) Goggles

28. How should soiled bed linens be handled?
  (A) By carrying them away from the nursing assistant's body
  (B) By shaking them in the air to get rid of contaminants
  (C) By taking them into another resident's room to put them in a hamper
  (D) By rolling them dirty side out

29. What is the purpose of the Health Insurance Portability and Accountability Act (HIPAA)?
  (A) To monitor quality of care in facilities
  (B) To reduce incidents of abuse in facilities
  (C) To keep protected health information private and secure
  (D) To provide training for facility staff

30. One safety device that helps transfer residents is called a
  (A) Waist restraint
  (B) Posey vest
  (C) Transfer belt
  (D) Geriatric chair

31. At which site is body temperature measured via the forehead?
  (A) Axillary
  (B) Tympanic
  (C) Temporal artery
  (D) Rectal

32. A nursing assistant should encourage a resident's independence and self-care because doing this
  (A) Promotes body function
  (B) Decreases blood flow
  (C) Lowers self-esteem
  (D) Increases anxiety

33. A restraint can be applied
  (A) When a resident is being rude to staff
  (B) When a nursing assistant does not have time to watch the resident
  (C) With a doctor's order
  (D) When a resident keeps pressing his call light

34. A nursing assistant can show she is listening carefully to a resident by
  (A) Looking away when the resident talks
  (B) Changing the subject often
  (C) Interrupting the resident to finish what he is saying
  (D) Focusing on the resident and giving feedback

35. How many milliliters equal one ounce?
  (A) 40
  (B) 30
  (C) 60
  (D) 20

36. With urinary catheters, it is important for a nursing assistant to remember that
  (A) Tubing should remain kinked and clean
  (B) Perineal care does not need to be performed
  (C) The drainage bag should be kept lower than the hips or the bladder
  (D) The tubing should be placed underneath the resident's body

37. When assisting a resident who has had a stroke, a nursing assistant should
  (A) Do everything for the resident
  (B) Lead with the stronger side when transferring
  (C) Dress the stronger side first
  (D) Place food in the weaker side of the mouth

38. In which stage is a dying resident if he insists that a mistake was made on his blood test and he is not really dying?
(A) Denial
(B) Bargaining
(C) Acceptance
(D) Depression

39. The process of helping to restore a person to her highest level of functioning is called
(A) Positioning
(B) Rehabilitation
(C) Elimination
(D) Retention

40. A nursing assistant overhears other nursing assistants discussing a resident. One of them says that she does not like taking care of this resident because "he is rude and smells funny." The nursing assistant should
(A) Join in the conversation and tell the others her opinion of this resident
(B) Let the resident know so that he will be nicer to the nursing assistants
(C) Suggest to the nursing assistants that this is not the place to have this discussion
(D) Ask another resident's opinion about how she should respond

41. An oral temperature should not be taken on a resident who has eaten or drunk fluids in the last _____ minutes.
(A) 25-35
(B) 10-20
(C) 40-50
(D) 50-60

42. How many feet does a quad cane have?
(A) 1
(B) 2
(C) 3
(D) 4

43. A nursing assistant can assist residents with their spiritual needs by
(A) Trying to convince residents to convert to the nursing assistant's religion
(B) Listening to residents talk about their beliefs
(C) Insisting residents participate in religious services
(D) Expressing judgments about residents' religious groups

44. When may a nursing assistant hit a resident?
(A) When the resident becomes combative
(B) When the resident threatens to hit the nursing assistant or someone else
(C) Only if the resident hits the nursing assistant first
(D) Never

45. When a resident has right-sided weakness, how should clothing be applied first?
(A) On the left side
(B) On the right side
(C) On whichever side is closer to the nursing assistant
(D) On whichever side the resident prefers

46. A resident offers a nursing assistant a gift for being such a good nursing assistant. The nursing assistant should
(A) Politely refuse the gift
(B) Politely accept the gift
(C) Accept the gift but donate it
(D) Ask the resident for money instead

47. According to the Omnibus Budget Reconciliation Act (OBRA), nursing assistants must complete at least ___ hours of training and must pass a competency evaluation before they can be employed.
(A) 100
(B) 250
(C) 50
(D) 75

48. Call lights should be placed
    (A) High on the wall over the head of the bed
    (B) Inside the bedside stand
    (C) On the floor
    (D) Within the resident's reach

49. How long should nursing assistants use friction when lathering and washing their hands?
    (A) 2 minutes
    (B) 5 seconds
    (C) 18 seconds
    (D) 20 seconds

50. The Occupational Safety and Health Administration (OSHA) is a federal government agency that protects workers from
    (A) Hazards on the job
    (B) Lawsuits
    (C) Workplace violence
    (D) Unfair employment practices